MENINGOENCEPHALITIS - DISEASE WHICH REQUIRES OPTIMAL APPROACH IN EMERGENCY MANNER

Edited by **Marina Pana**

Meningoencephalitis - Disease Which Requires Optimal Approach in Emergency Manner
http://dx.doi.org/10.5772/63137
Edited by Marina Pana

Contributors

Masaraf Hussain, Franc Strle, Petra Bogovič, Sandip Kumar Dash, Jean-Paul Gonzalez, Sergey Kramarev, Hennadii A. Mokhort, Marina Pana

Published by InTech
Janeza Trdine 9, 51000 Rijeka, Croatia

Notice

Publishing Process Manager Dajana Pemac
Technical Editor SPi Global
Cover InTech Design team

First published August, 2017
Printed in Croatia
Legal deposit, Croatia: National and University Library in Zagreb

Additional hard copies can be obtained from orders@intechopen.com

Meningoencephalitis - Disease Which Requires Optimal Approach in Emergency Manner, Edited by Marina Pana
p. cm.
Print ISBN 978-953-51-3471-8
Online ISBN 978-953-51-3472-5

For EU product safety concerns:
IN TECH d.o.o., Prolaz Marije Krucifikse Kozulić 3, 51000 Rijeka, Croatia,
info@intechopen.com or visit our website at intechopen.com.

Meet the editor

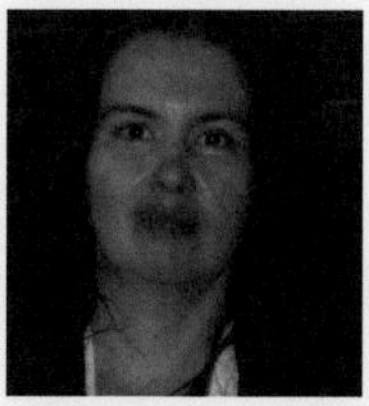

Marina Pana, MD, PhD, RS II, works at Cantacuzino National Research Institute, being the head of Vaccine-Preventable Diseases lab. From 2008, she has been appointed as operational contact point for the European Centre for Disease Prevention and Control (ECDC), regarding S. pneumoniae and N. meningitidis, two main agents involved in meningitis etiology.

During her career, Dr. Pana has contributed to a number of workshops and medical seminars as their coordinator as well as lecturer. She has attended numerous European congresses (oral communications) especially those concerning pneumococci and meningococci involved in invasive infections and also published several works on bacterial agents that caused meningitis. Dr. Pana is a reviewer of Romanian and international journals and member of the ESCMID and European Society of Chemotherapy (ESC).

Contents

Preface

Meningoencephalitis remains a major global threat, despite the prevention, diagnosis, and antibiotic therapy that have been improved considerably in the last years.

The diagnostic approach urgently established, etiologic agent identified, and empirical antimicrobial therapy remain a continuous challenge, especially in immunocompromised patients.

In this thematic issue, the scientists present their results of accomplished studies, in order to provide several guidelines regarding the strategies of diagnosis and treatment of patients with meningoencephalitis.

The guidelines are necessarily asked, and those using the guidelines are advised to seek expert advice on the management of cases (from clinical microbiologists, infectious disease physicians, infection control, public health physicians, and occupational health physicians) as required. The guidance can be adapted depending on local circumstances and risk assessment of each suspected case or situation and will contribute to a considerable progress in medical field.

However, meningoencephalitis remains a public health concern and continues to claim many lives, despite the availability of potent antibiotics. Any delay in the diagnosis of this illness could cause morbidity and death.

I take this occasion to thank so much all the contributors of this book, who played a critical role in gathering data for public health decision, with precision, perseverance, and dedication, adding valuable data and completing our knowledge regarding some meningoencephalitis aspects.

Dr. Marina Pana
Head of Vaccine-Preventable Diseases Lab
Operational Contact Point for S. pneumoniae and N. meningitidis for ECDC
"Cantacuzino" National Research Institute
Bucharest, Romania

Chapter 1

Introductory Chapter: Meningoencephalitis

Marina Pana

Additional information is available at the end of the chapter

http://dx.doi.org/10.5772/intechopen.70366

1. Introduction

Meningitis continues to claim many lives, despite the availability of potent antibiotics to destroy the deadly pathogens. Acute bacterial meningitis (ABM) is an uncommon but potentially fatal neurologic emergency that requires prompt recognition, diagnostic evaluation, and initiation of parenteral antibiotics [1]. Bacterial meningitis is very serious and can be deadly. Death can occur in as little as a few hours.

Common causes of bacterial meningitis vary by age group (newborns, babies and children, teens and young adults, older adults). And certain people are at increased risk for bacterial meningitis, those including: age, community setting, certain medical conditions, working with meningitis-causing pathogens, and travel [1].

It is very important to highlight the clinical overlap between encephalitis and meningo encephalitis.

The diagnosis becomes challenging when patients present with nonspecific clinical features. Meningitis results from inflammation of the pia-arachnoid meninges as well as cerebrospinal fluid [2, 3]. Encephalitis refers to inflammation of the brain parenchyma and is typically characterized by cognitive deficits. Of the pathogens reported to cause encephalitis, the majority are viruses.

However, despite extensive testing, the etiology of encephalitis remains unknown in most patients. Another major challenge for patients with encephalitis is to determine the relevance of an infectious agent identified outside of the CNS; these agents may play a role in the neurologic manifestations of illness but not necessarily by directly invading the CNS. In addition, it is important to distinguish between infectious encephalitis and post infectious or post immunization encephalitis, encephalomyelitis [e.g., acute disseminated encephalomyelitis (ADEM)], which may be mediated by an immunologic response to an antecedent antigenic stimulus from an infecting microorganism or immunization [4].

It is important to realize that guidelines cannot always account for individual variation among patients. They are not intended to supplant physician judgment with respect to particular patients or special clinical situations. The Infectious Diseases Society of America considers adherence to these guidelines to be voluntary, with the ultimate determination regarding their application to be made by the physician in the light of each patient's individual circumstances [4].

The clinical distinction between meningitis and encephalitis is frequently blurred as patients often present with signs and symptoms of both conditions. These patients can best be described as having meningoencephalitis, the pathologic condition that results when inflammation spreads from the CSF and meninges to the adjacent brain parenchyma [1]. Inflammation of the central nervous system can be acute, subacute, or chronic in duration and community, or nosocomial in origin. Although meningeal inflammation may be due to medications, neoplastic or autoimmune processes, or nonbacterial microbes (e.g., viruses, fungi, or parasites), bacterial infection remains the most studied cause.

The existing literature on ABM is limited in several ways. First, much of the research on the pathophysiology of meningitis has been based on experimental rabbit and rat models. Second, much of our current understanding about the clinical features, diagnosis, and prognosis of ABM has been extracted from chart reviews. These reviews rarely report methodology and are heavily dependent on the availability and accuracy of the medical records. Furthermore, because reviewers cannot adequately control for confounding variables, the retrospective data cannot be used to establish cause-effect relationships; only potential associations between variables can be pointed out. Third, a good number of trials involving bacterial etiology and therapy have been conducted in the international setting. In general, the results of these studies cannot be extrapolated to practice within the United States. The external validity of all studies must be assessed before a new treatment strategy can be adopted [1].

It is always very important to distinguish community-acquired bacterial meningitis from encephalitis, aseptic meningitis, and intracranial abscess.

Microbiologists play a critical role in gathering data both for clinical and public health decision making [5]. Thus, high-quality surveillance, including molecular methods and fine typing, is crucial to accurately detect and assess changes in the epidemiology of bacteria (e.g., invasive meningococcal disease) and ensure sufficient understanding of the need for, and impact and effectiveness of, vaccination [5].

The priority of the vaccine and how it can be integrated into the national immunization program are also important to consider [6]. Considering these factors, the cost effectiveness and feasibility of introducing a new vaccine needs to be based on country-specific assessments [7].

Author details

Marina Pana

Address all correspondence to: marina.pana@yahoo.com

National Research Institute "Cantacuzino", Bucharest, Romania

References

[1] Sadoun T, Singh A. Adult acute bacterial meningitis in the United States: 2009 update. Emergency Medicine Practice. EB Medicine. 2009;11(9)

[2] McCracken GH, Sande MA, Lentnek A, Whitley RJ, Scheld WM. Evaluation of new anti-infective drugs for the treatment of acute bacterial meningitis. Infectious Disease Society of America and the Food and Drug Administration. Clinical Infectious Disease. 1992;15(Suppl 1):S182-S188

[3] Overturf GD. Defining bacterial meningitis and other infections of the central nervous system. Pediatric Critical Care Medicine. 2005;6(3 Suppl):S14-S18

[4] Tunkel AR, Glaser CA, Bloch KC, Sejvar JJ, Marra CM, Roos KL, Hartman BJ, Kaplan SL, Scheld WM, Whitley RJ. The management of encephalitis: Clinical practice guidelines by the infectious diseases Society of America. Clinical Infectious Diseases. 2008;47:303-327. DOI: 10.1086/589747

[5] Whittacker R, Dias JG, Ramliden M, Kodmon C, Economopoulou A, Beer N, Pastore CL, The ECDC Network Members for Invasive Meningococcal Disease. The epidemiology of invasive meningococcal disease in EU/EEA countries 2004-2014. Vaccine. 2017;35:2034-2041.

[6] Trotter CL, Ramsay ME. Vaccination against meningococcal disease in Europe: Review and recommendations for the use of conjugate vaccines. FEMS Microbiology Reviews. 2007, January;31(1):101-107

[7] Takla A, et al. Characteristics and practices of National Immunization Technical Advisory groups in Europe and potential for collaboration. April 2014. Euro Surveillance. 2015;20:9

Chapter 2

Biosurveillance of Meningococcal Infection in Ukraine, 43 Years of Survey: Spatial and Temporal Dynamics Models

Hennadii Mokhort, Sergey Kramarev and Jean-Paul J. Gonzalez

Additional information is available at the end of the chapter

http://dx.doi.org/10.5772/intechopen.68371

Abstract

Meningococcal disease in Ukraine represents an important cause of mortality mostly among the child population of less than five-year old. The present study illustrates the advancement on understanding of Meningococcal epidemiology across the national level by using20 years of data provided by the Ministry of Health of Ukraine on a constant survey of the disease. This unique set of data includes: demography (census); disease incidence from 1973 to 2015 (i.e., purulent meningitis etiologic diagnostic); Meningococcal disease mortality; anonymized demographic data (sex, age, leaving area/city/village); Comparative etiology of purulent meningitis; serogroups of invasive meningococcal disease; carriers prevalence; a set of clinical data (meningitis, meningococcemia, nasopharyngitis, etc.); and a set of environmental data (season, etc.). The dynamic of the disease is described for over the past 20-year period of time including incidence, prevalence, spatial distribution, seasonality, and risk factors. Existing state of the art of meningococcal infection epidemiology is presented for the all country. Ultimately, time series analysis of record and spatial distribution over such a long period of time supported the development of original construct of various models encompassing risk and vulnerability, and ways to improve epidemiological surveillance, and develop vaccination strategies in country.

Keywords: meningitis, meningococcemia, time series, modeling, Ukraine

1. Introduction

1.1. Background

To date, purulent bacterial meningitis (PBM) remains a global health challenge. Meningococcal meningitis occurs in small clusters throughout the World with seasonal variation, accounts for a variable proportion of epidemic bacterial meningitis, and is one of the leading causes of such meningitis globally with a burden that, in 2012 encompassed 395,230 deaths, or 0.7% of global mortality [1, 2].

Meningococcal disease or meningococcal meningitis is caused by bacterium *Neisseria meningitidis*, also called meningococcus. Meningococcal bacteria may cause infection, which occurs in different compartment of the body, called invasive meningococcal disease (IMD), including skin, gastrointestinal tract, or respiratory tract, among others. Ultimately, the bacteria may pass through the bloodstream and reach the nervous system causing meningococcal meningitis. After an incubation period of 2–10 days, clinical presentation starts with symptoms similar to influenza (flu-like), which cause nausea, vomiting, rash, increased sensitivity to light, and confusion. Symptoms of meningococcal disease appear usually as a sudden onset of fever, headache, and stiff neck. When treated, most patients with meningococcal meningitis recover completely with appropriate antibiotic therapy and rapid medical attention. Also, meningitis can cause severe brain damage and be fatal for 50% of untreated cases.

There is no animal reservoir, and *N. meningitidis* is obligate commensals of human and can colonize the nasopharyngeal mucosa without affecting the host, a phenomenon known as carriage. Such asymptomatic carriage of meningococcus is the most prevalent form of meningococcal infection. In none-epidemic settings, approximately 10–35% of healthy individuals carry *N. meningitidis* in the upper airway [3, 4]. Thus, only in very rare cases, *N. meningitidis* is the cause of invasive meningococcal disease. *N. meningitidis* is transmitted from person-to-person through respiratory droplets or throat secretions from carriers or eventually patients. The risk of transmission and spread increases in particular by close and prolonged contact (e.g., kissing, sneezing, coughing, promiscuity, and sharing food or drinking utensils) with an infected person (symptomatic or asymptomatic (i.e., carrier). Moreover, such risk increases with recent upper respiratory infection, while young children and teen-agers are at greatest risk of infection.

Several types of meningococcal vaccines are available including Meningococcal Polysaccharide vaccines as bivalent (groups A and C), trivalent (groups A, C and W), or tetravalent (groups A, C, Y and W). Tetravalent A, C, Y, and W conjugate vaccines have been licensed since 2005 for use in children and adults in Canada, the United States of America, and Europe. Since 1999, meningococcal conjugate vaccines against group C have been available and widely used. (e.g., Meningococcal conjugate vaccine; Meningococcal polysaccharide vaccine; Serogroup B Meningococcal B) and are recommended vaccines as the best that can prevent meningitis infection. As of June 2015, over 220 million persons aged 1–29-year old received meningococcal A conjugate vaccine against the most meningitis type prevalent among 15 countries of the African belt [2].

http://dx.doi.org/10.5772/intechopen.68371

1.2. Epidemic pattern of Meningococcal meningitis in Europe

There is a reported reduction of morbidity of Invasive Meningococcal Disease (IMD) in the European countries (i.e., EU/EEA): The total number of confirmed cases of the IMD fell from 7995 to 3463 for the period from 1999 to 2012. In countries with a meningococcal serogroup C vaccination program, the number of cases fell from 4840 to 2380, in countries where systematic immunization campaigns are not applied incidence decreased from 3155 cases to 1083 cases [5, 6]. Therefore, a reduction of IMD mortality in EU/EEA countries was reported that diminished from 0.163 to 0.055 per 100,000 people from 1992 to 2012 [7]. Although, IMD is relatively rare in Europe (0.68 cases/100,000 people in 2012), country-specific rates of confirmed IMD range from 0.11 to 1.77 cases per 100,000 people [8].

Worldwide, most IMD cases are caused by serogroups B and C. Serogroup Y prevalence has been increasing but remains less frequent than B and C. An overall decreasing trend has been observed over the last 10 years, partly attributable to the introduction of serogroup C conjugate vaccine to national immunization schedules in several European countries.

Finally, it is of importance to strengthen surveillance of meningococcal disease in order to reduce burden of the disease (including patient and carrier) and to evaluate the impact of the ongoing vaccination programs, and support decision-makers with respect to the availability of new vaccines [6].

2. Meningococcal infection biosurveillance and Public Health response and control in Ukraine

The purpose of epidemiological surveillance of meningococcal infection (MI) is to prevent deaths and reduce disease morbidity risk groups. A retrospective epidemiological analysis of MI must include data monitoring morbidity risk groups (e.g., children aged of 0–1 and 1–4 years old), and other young people as which came as socio-organized as group indicators (i.e., including school, kindergartens, orphanages, vocational colleges, university, among others). Equally important is the analysis of total mortality and mortality by risk groups and their dynamics. In addition, data are analyzed from microbiological monitoring of "indicator groups." Moreover, there is a national serological monitoring of MI pathogens.

In epidemic foci of MI, patients with IMD are hospitalized and isolated while and a 10 days' medical observation of contact-persons is conducted (thermometry and examination of the skin and mucous membranes of the nasopharynx). Bacteriological tests are done twice among organized groups and once at home (i.e., family contact) within epidemic foci. Surveillance of other purulent meningitis is carried out as for meningococcal infection.

In Ukraine, since the 1920s, MI cases introduced are registered as well as *Haemophilus influenzae* type B Hib-meningitis cases are registered since 2010. From 2012, pneumococcal meningitis (PM) and all other bacterial meningitis are also registered. Vaccination against Hib-infection was included in the routine immunization program in 2006 by the Ministry of Health, while it is considering now to introduce a national vaccination campaigns against meningococcal and pneumococcal disease. As of 2013, an estimated of 68.9% of Ukrainians lives in urban areas including the 68.2% of the population over 45 years old [8].

Since 2007, there is a Central Reference Laboratory for invasive bacterial diseases (IBD) characterizing and supervising the dynamic of IBD pathogens in order to forecast and reduce (preventive measures) the incidence of IBD. The State institution "Ukrainian Centre for Disease Control and monitoring of the Ministry of Health of Ukraine" is a reference as part of the IBD-laboratory WHO and UNICEF networks. A sentinel surveillance system included all patients younger than 5 years clinically suspected of meningitis and hospitalized as hospital in-patient of either the department of infectious disease or intensive care unit.

3. Temporal and spatialdynamics of meningococcal infection in Ukraine

3.1. Place and time of meningococcal infection and other purulent meningitis

Purulent bacterial meningitis (PBM) is a group of diseases of multi-bacterial etiology that determines the nature of the treatment, laboratory diagnostic approach and epidemiological characteristics for control and prevention. Indeed, PBM transmission and clinical presentation are fully dependent on the etiologic agent and concurrent risk factor. PBM etiology will ensure a successful causal treatment and important information regarding the whole nosology of the meningitis and epidemiology pattern. Bacteriological etiological diagnosis of PBM has been carried out for 24 years (1992–2015) in Ukraine (Ukrainian Centre for Disease Control and monitoring of the Ministry of Health): 37,843 cases were registered as PBM, among them, 18,878 were of purulent meningitis of meningococcal origin and other IMD. The ratio of meningococcal meningitis to non-meningococcal meningitis was about more or less of 1:1 (i.e., 49.89 to 50.11%) (**Figure 1**).

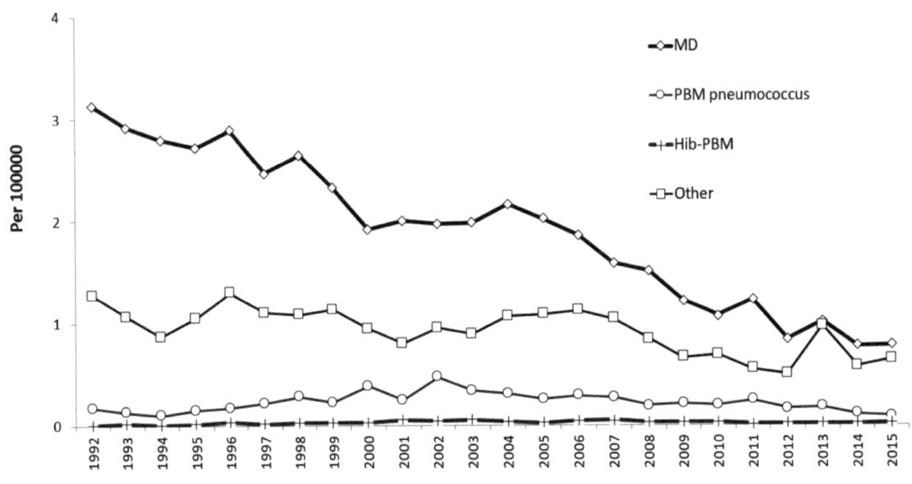

Figure 1. Incidence dynamics of different etiological forms of bacterial meningitis (Ukraine, 1992–2015). Legend: Abscissa = time (year); Ordinate = case of bacterial meningitis per 100,000 people; Empty diamond = Meningococcal Disease (MD); Empty square = Other Meningitis (caused by *Staphylococcus aureus, Streptococcus* groups A and B, *Klebsiella pneumoniae, Escherichia coli, Listeria monocytogenes* and PBM of unknown etiology); Empty circle = PBM pneumococcus (Purulent Bacterial Meningitis caused by *Streptococcus pneumonia*); Cross = Haemophilus influenzae type b (Hib).

The use of microbiological monitoring of PBM in Ukraine allowed to determine the etiological origin of 37,843 cases from 1992 to 2012. The basic etiological agents PBM included: Meningococci (49.89%); Pneumococci (6.34%); Staphylococci, Streptococci and others (*Escherichia* spp., *Listeria* spp., etc.) (17.30%); Hib-infection (0.71%), and pathogens of unknown etiology (25.77%). Among the 21,359 registered cases of MI, 9986 cases (46.75%) were confirmed to be of bacteriological origin. Bacteriological confirmation of MI ranges from 33.71% in 1993 to 55.95% 9 years after (2002) (**Figure 2**).

Meningococcal infection predominated among all bacterial meningitis during the whole period of observation. However, half of all non-meningococcal meningitis as well as IMD did not have bacteriological confirmation the bacteriological tests were done almost in all patients but were not positive for half of all meningococcal meningitis. Thus, the total sensitivity of bacteriological tests was inadequate (nearly 50%).

3.2. Time series of morbidity and mortality of meningococcal infection in Ukraine

In 1969, an incidence of less than 0.9 per 100,000 people of MI was recorded. Since then, the incidence began to rise and lasted until 1985. For decade (1973–2012), MI incidence (including all clinical forms) ranged from 6.7 (1985) to 0.83 (2012) per 100,000 people. Instead, in the long term, of IMD and mortality appear be very specific and different dynamics, while IMD incidence is much lower and ranges from 2.22 (1974) to 0.75 (2012) per 100,000 people with a mortality from 0.84 (1983) to 0.09 (**Figure 3**).

There is a significant decrease morbidity and mortality of MI for the last 33 years in Ukraine. Between 1983 and 2015 the incidence of MI decreased by 7.2 times. Between 1973 and 2015

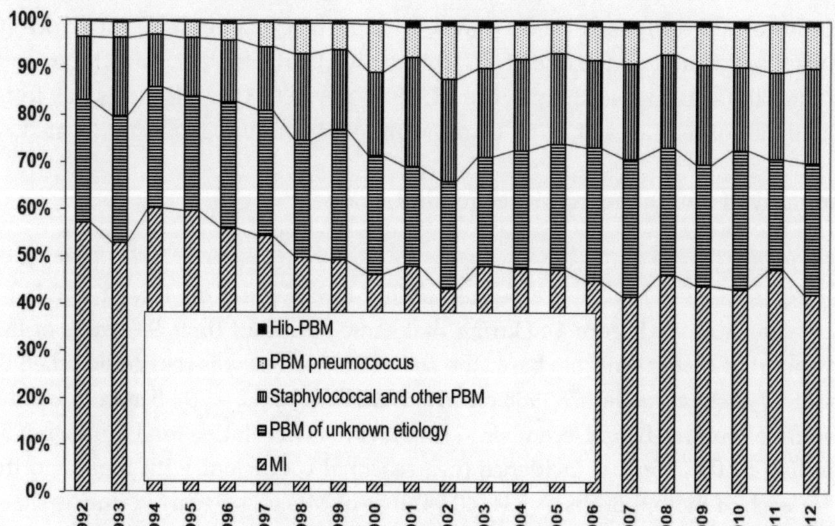

Figure 2. Etiological structure of purulent meningitis cases in Ukraine (1992–2012). Legend: Abscissa = Time (year); Ordinate = relative percentage of the bacterial meningitis etiology; oblique lines = Meningococcal Infection (MI); vertical lines = Staphylococcal and Other PBM (caused by *Staphylococcus aureus, Streptococcus* groups A and B, *Klebsiella pneumoniae, Escherichia coli, Listeria monocytogenes* and other PBM); horizontal lines = PBM of unknown etiology); points = PBM pneumococcus (Purulent Bacterial Meningitis caused by *Streptococcus pneumoniae*); black = *Haemophilus influenzae* type b (Hib-PBM).

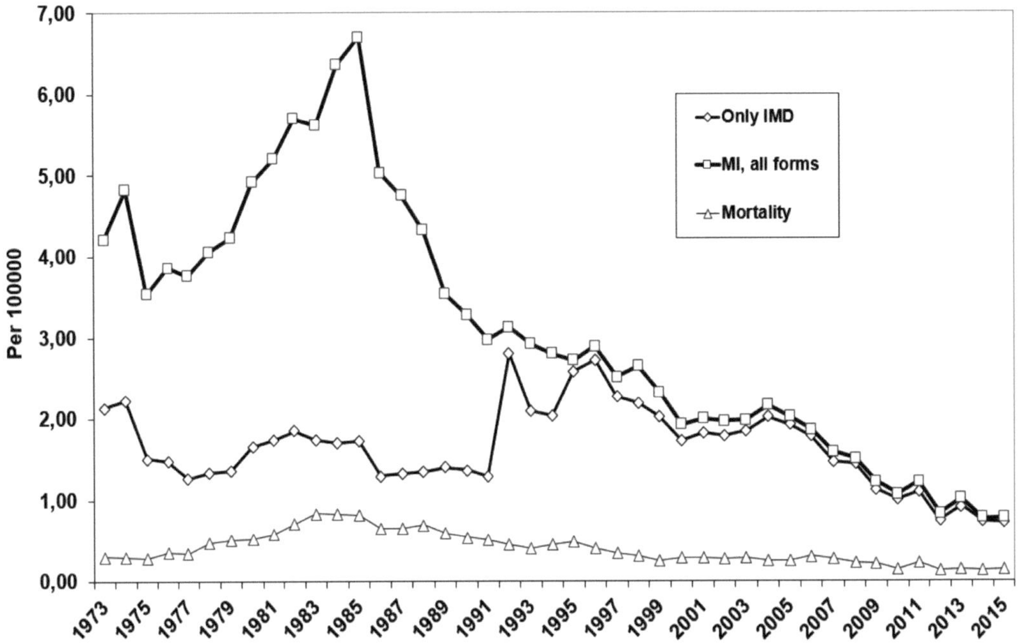

Figure 3. Morbidity and mortality dynamics of meningococcal infection in Ukraine of a decade of observation (1973–2015). Legend: Abscissa = time (year); Ordinate = patient meningococcal infection per 100,000 people; line with empty square = Meningococcal Infection (total MI, all clinic forms); line with empty diamond = Invasive Meningococcal Disease (IMD); line with empty triangle = total Mortality of Meningococcal Infection.

the incidence of MI decreased by 5.4 times. In 2012 in Ukraine, IMD incidence (0.75 per 100,000) was comparable to the one of EU (0.7 per 100,000). However, death rate in Ukraine (0.09 per 100,000) was higher than in the EU (0.06 per 100,000). Also, this has to take into account that half of the cases of MI in Ukraine are not bacteriologically confirmed.

3.3. Seasonality of meningococcal infection in Ukraine

From 1992 to 2015, most IMD cases occurred in winter and spring, as for other respiratory diseases in Ukraine. IMD incidence peaked up in March, while the lowest number of cases was reported in August (**Figure 4**). During that same period of time, 938 cases of IMD were regularly reported on the monthly base, and seasonal increase was registered when the number of monthly cases exceeded 78 (938 cases / 12 month = 78.2 ≈ 78). Seasonal incidence rise was lasted for 6 months (from December to June) with a cumulative total number of 554 cases corresponding 59.06% annual incidence (i.e., seasonal coefficient with regard to the 9.84% average for each of these months. A 334 (40.94%) as of MI cases occurred during the seasonal rise with a monthly increase of 6.82%. One can ultimately evaluate the cases associated with seasonal risk factors that were in 18.66%, i.e. (9.84% – 6.82%) × 6 months = 18.66%.

Thus, the impact of seasonal factors on the annual incidence is very moderate, that is, annual incidence of MI is due to the seasonality of not more than one-fifth of part. Over 80% of

http://dx.doi.org/10.5772/intechopen.68371

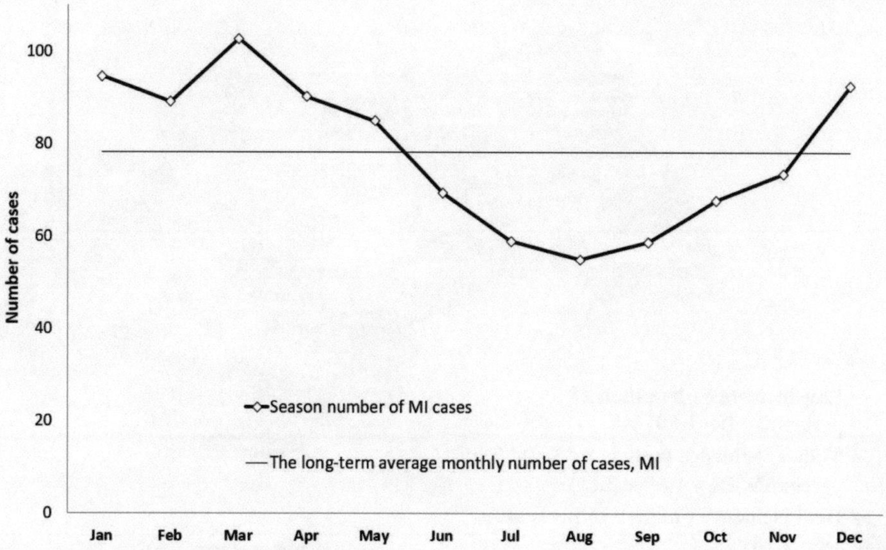

Figure 4. Seasonal distribution of meningococcal infection in Ukraine (1992–2015). Legend: Abscissa = time (months); Ordinate = absolute number of cases of meningococcal infection; Gray line = the average monthly number of Meningococcal Infection (MI) cases of long-term; Empty diamond = number of Meningococcal Infection (MI) cases by month.

incidence of MI depends on the action of permanent factors. Our hypothesis is that the proportion of susceptible population and the frequency of contacts between people (at risk of infection) are the basic are a permanent risk of MI transmission. We also assume that its values are slightly slowly changing throughout the year. Such seasonal rise was observed in Europe from December to June is also characterized by a seasonality pattern as it is in Ukraine, with the highest rate reporting during winter [8].

3.4. Geographical distribution

The incidence of MI is unevenly distributed on a geographical ground and expressed by ANOVA MI incidence for the 1992–2013 period of times among administrative units of Ukraine. Estimated value (Fisher's test = 8.52, > critical value of 1.52) rejects the null hypothesis of no effect of geographical factors on the incidence of MI. Indeed, **Figure 5** shows the uneven geographical distribution of the disease by administrative units with low, medium, and high levels of incidence.

At first, the geographical distribution of MI incidence depends on population age pyramid including, the total population of the study area, the urban population and the child population of 0–14 or 0–4-year old. We therefore calculated the corresponding correlation coefficients, but ultimately lacked of statistical significance between prevalence and administrative units. MI incidence correlation coefficients, when compared to different group, were equal to: 0.3260 versus population density; 0.036 versus total population; 0.1711 versus urban population percentage; 0.1370 versus children aged 0–14; and 0.1968 versus the children aged

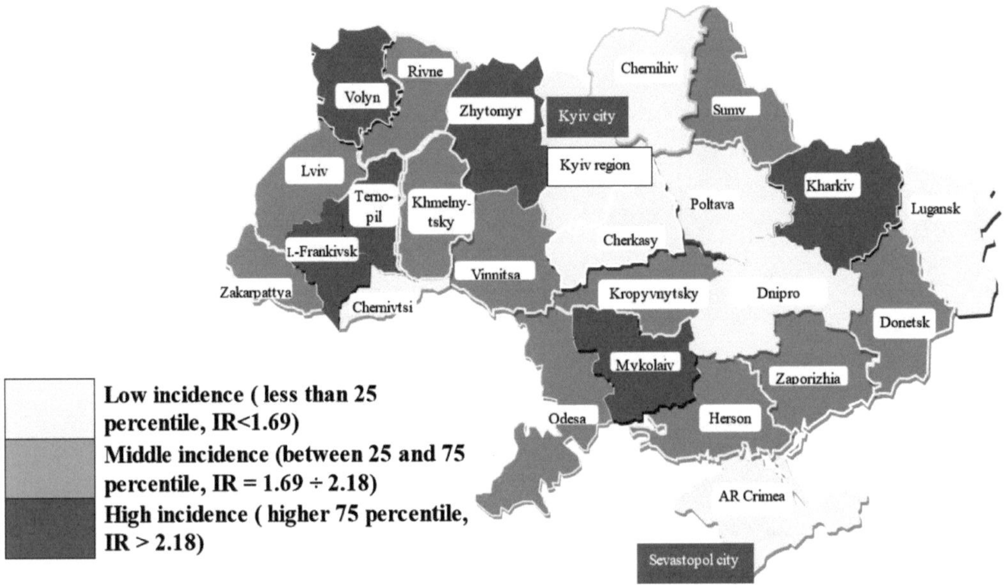

Figure 5. Incidence of meningococcal disease in Ukraine by oblast (1992–2013). Legend: light-gray = Low incidence of Meningococcal Disease (less than 25 percentiles, IR<1.69); moderately gray = Middle incidence of Meningococcal Disease (between 25 and 75 percentile, IR = 1.69 ÷ 2.18); gray = High incidence of Meningococcal Disease (higher 75 percentile, IR > 2.18).

0–4 years. We believe that the lack of statistical significance between these indicators suggest sporadic (or random) spatial nature distribution of the disease. Also, ANOVA analysis shows significant differences in the incidence among oblasts, but the correlation analysis of individual factors (population density, age structure, etc.) by oblasts did not show any incidence because the population density and age structure are indirect factors. Thus, we can assume that geographical factors of each individual territory are quite stable, while geography has a limited effect on changes in incidence of MI in Ukraine. Geographical distribution of MI incidence is useful for comparing performance in different areas, but it cannot account for observed differences more likely linked to the multicomponent result with other causal factors. Also, the variable power of causal factors in any oblast could explain the differences in the incidence oblasts. In our case, the geographical distribution of the incidence of MI is a little informative because do not allowed to identify direct factors (i.e., risk of infection and/or risk of susceptibility).

3.5. Age distribution

The total incidence of MI decreased over the study period in Ukraine among all age groups, while it remains the highest among young children (**Figure 6**).

In Ukraine, the proportion of MI infected children under 14 years represented 77.17% of all cases as compared to 49.81% among the same xc of age of other European countries at

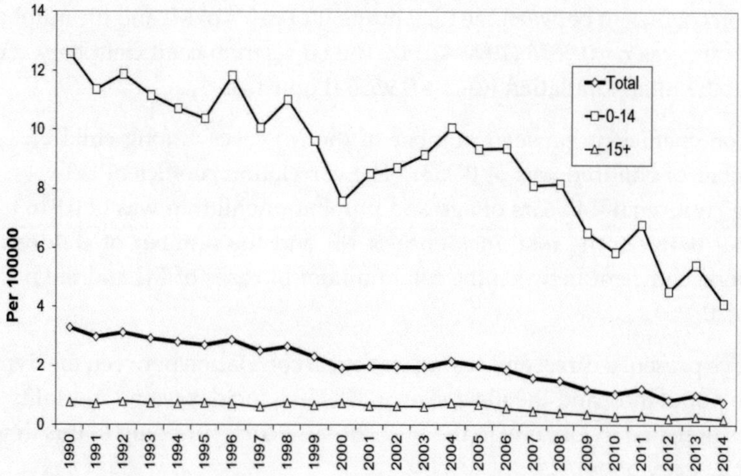

Figure 6. Dynamics of the incidence of meningococcal infection in Ukraine by age group (1990–2014). Legend: Abscissa = time (year); Ordinate = person with meningococcal infection per 100,000 people by age group; Triangle = Incidence of Meningococcal Disease among the population aged over 15 years; Square = Incidence of Meningococcal Disease among children aged 0-14 years; Diamond = Incidence of Meningococcal Disease among the total population.

large [8]. Thus, children under 14 years in Ukraine are at a major risk for MI infection, and mortality rates account for 78.35% (**Figure 7**). Altogether, there is a strong direct relationship of MI incidence among age groups that exactly fit the local pyramid of age.

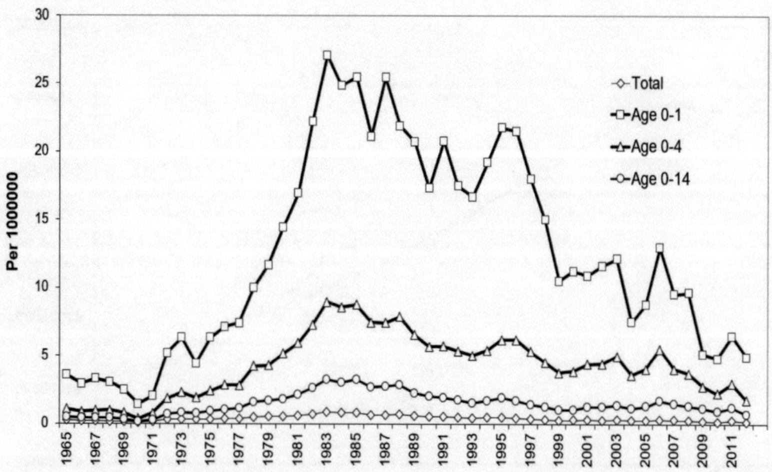

Figure 7. Mortality of meningococcal infectious disease among you children by class of age (Ukraine, 1965–2012). Legend: Legend: Abscissa = time (year); Ordinate = person with meningococcal infection per 100,000 people by age class; Empty circle = Incidence of Meningococcal Disease among children aged 0-14 years; Square = Incidence of Meningococcal Disease among children aged 0-1 years; Diamond = Incidence of Meningococcal Disease among the total population; Triangle = Incidence of Meningococcal Disease among children aged 0-4 years.

The correlation coefficient between the total number of cases of MI and the number of population for the years was r = 0.9676 (1990–2014). The correlation coefficient between the overall incidence and the total population was r = 0.9556 (**Figure 8**).

The correlation coefficient between number of the MI cases among children 0–14 years of age and number of children was of 0.9531. The correlation coefficient between the MI incidence among children 0–14 years of age and number of children was of 0.8163. The correlation coefficient between the total incidence of MI and the number of children was 0.9239. The correlation coefficient between the total number of cases of MI and the number of children was 0.9420.

All of the above present a direct and strong statistical correlation between the dynamics of age structure, the population and the incidence of MI. Peak incidence and mortality of meningococcal disease occurred in Ukraine in the mid-80s, also corresponding to this time of national birth rates or a "baby boom."

Children's age is an indirect risk factor for invasive meningococci disease (IMD), while youngest children are more susceptibility to the pathogen, including predisposing factor of IMD and high transmission risk among over-crowded communities (i.e., school, recreation area, etc.). Incidence may also be reduced when the relative number of children decreases, and the whole population is aging (as it is in Ukraine and Europe). Indeed, during the study period, the number of children relatively decreased by twofold among general population, while the total number of population also decreased in Ukraine. Thus, we believe that the incidence of IMD in different age groups defined different levels of susceptibility of the pathogen for these groups.

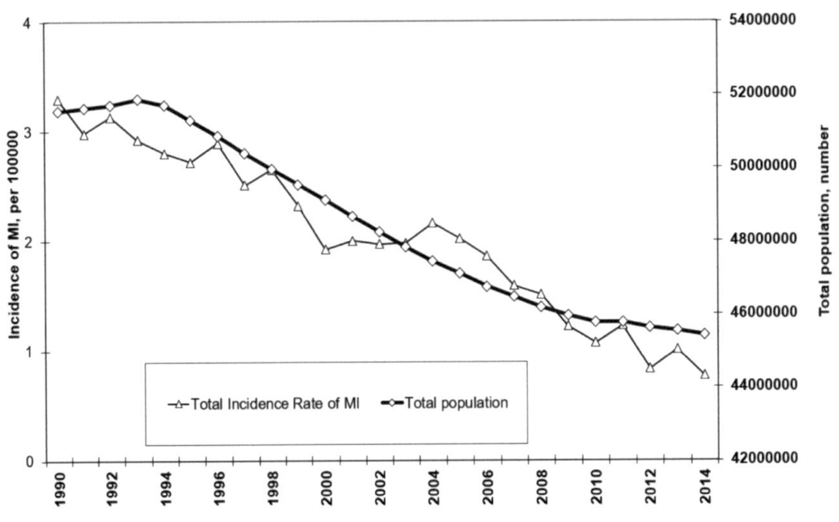

Figure 8. The dynamics of relationship between the overall incidence of meningococcal infection and the general population (Ukraine, 1990–2014). Legend: Abscissa = time (year); Ordinate = case of meningococcal infection per 100,000 people; Diamond = number of the total population; Triangle = Incidence of Meningococcal Disease among the total population.

3.6. Spatial rural as compared to urban distribution of meningococcal infection

In **Figure 9**, we see that the frequency of MI between cities and villages differ slightly. In cities, the total number and density of the population is greater than in the villages. This is evidenced by the result of ANOVA analysis of MI incidence for the period of 1990–2014 years for the urban and rural population of Ukraine. Estimated value of Fisher criterion (1.2) is less than the critical value (4.04). Thus, we have confirmed the statistical null hypothesis of no effect of residence on the incidence of MI.

These data may indicate that the percentage of the susceptible population in cities and towns are approximately equal. He also points to the sporadic incidence of MI in Ukraine.

3.7. Meningococcal carriage

Indeed, as a first factor in favor of such observations, one has to consider that meningococcus carriage is the most widespread form of meningococcal infection, that is, for one patient with IMD there is an estimate of more than thousands asymptomatic carriers of the pathogen. Carriage rates can range between 1 and 50% while varies with age, socioeconomic status, and connected with the predominant strain circulating in the area, and a number that appears not to vary with season or herd immunity. However, nasopharyngeal carriage surveillance is not recommended neither reported as a practical useful public health tool [9]. Also, data on nasopharyngeal carriage are available from state bacteriological laboratory in Ukraine (Ukrainian Centre for Disease Control and monitoring of the Ministry of Health of Ukraine) (**Figure 10**). Indeed, diagnostic tests are run annually by the Sanitary-epidemiological service

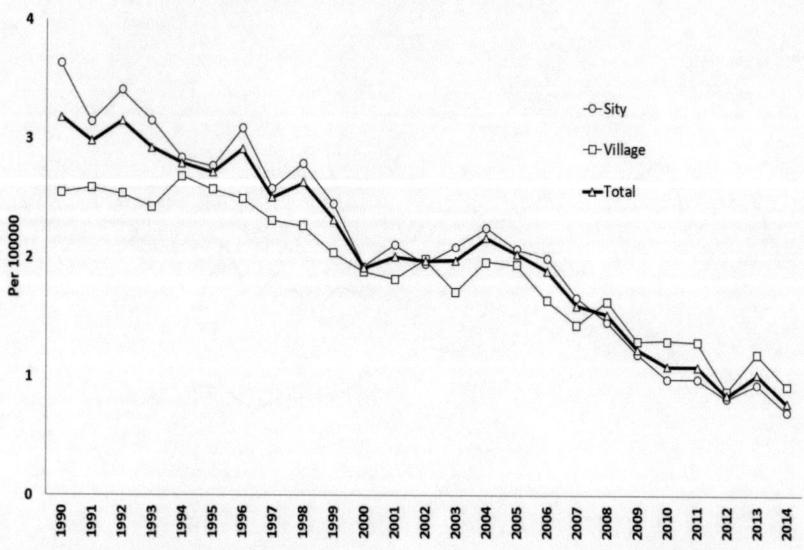

Figure 9. Dynamics of meningococcal infection in Ukraine in rural and urban areas (1990–2014). Legend: Abscissa = time (year); Ordinate = case of meningococcal infection per 100,000 people; Circle = Incidence of Meningococcal Disease in urban settings; Square = Incidence of Meningococcal Disease in rural; Triangle = Incidence of Meningococcal Disease among total population.

of Ukraine using nasopharyngeal swab. This approach was conducted in order to identify the level of circulating *N. meningitidis* in Ukraine among the healthy children and adolescents and also among all persons who had contact with MI patients, while contact persons represent all age groups or the general population. Such study was carried out in all 26 regions (oblasts) of Ukraine.

From 1992 to 2012, 890,061 people (average of 42,384/year) were investigated, moreover, 482,435 healthy people (average of 23,973/year) of all ages who have had contact with confirmed patients with MI, were also tested for meningococcal carriage in Ukraine. The results of these time series of MI carriers are shown in **Figure 9** and show the risk among healthy children and adolescents as an average of 0.99% as compared to 1.97% of the general population. Ultimately, such risk of infection is a factor of emergence of IMD and determines the level of prevalence of a small percentage of carriers is due to the large stratum of old adults and the low sensitivity of bacterial tests in Ukraine. The risk of infection is a necessary susceptibility factor for the emergence of IMI and therefore constantly determines the level of prevalence of meningococcal carriage.

3.8. Meningococcus serogroup distribution

In 1992–2012, information on the meningococcus serogroups was reported for 9484 IMD cases in Ukraine. The meningococcus B serogroup was responsible for 48.9% of IMD, followed by the meningococcus A serogroup (15.78%) and the meningococcus C serogroup (13.21%). The meningococcus D, X, Y, Z, 29E and W135 made up to 3.19% of IMD cases. Non-capsular strains represented 18.91%. During that same period, total information on serogroup was reported for 15,868 carriers. The meningococcus serogroup B was responsible for 36.15%

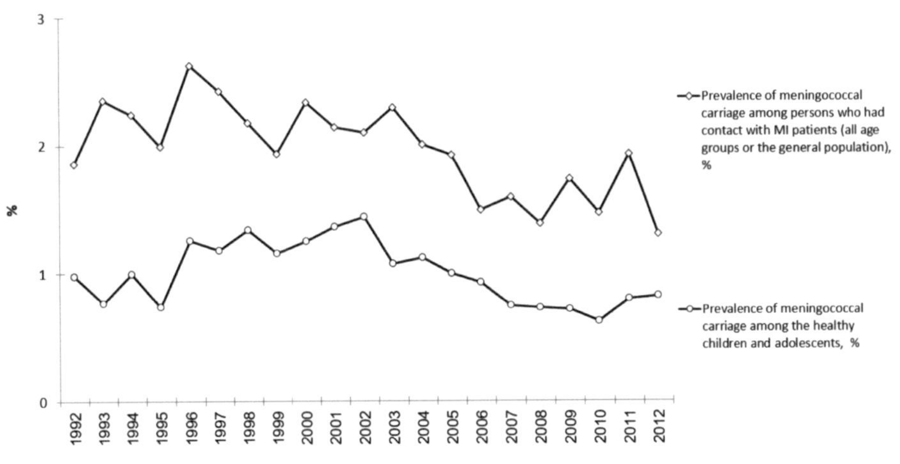

Figure 10. Meningococcal carriage dynamics among different population group survey in Ukraine (1992–2012). Legend: Abscissa = time (year); Ordinate = absolute number of carriers of meningococci; Circle = Prevalence (%) of meningococcal carriage among the healthy children and adolescents; Diamond = Prevalence (%) of meningococcal carriage among persons who had contact with MI patients (all age groups or the general population).

of carriers of meningococcal infections, followed by serogroup C (7.74%) and serogroup A (7.17%). The meningococcus serogroups D, X, Y, Z, 29E and W135 represented 6.75% of carriers' meningococcal infections the known serogroup. Not typed strain represented 42.19% of carriers of meningococcal infections (**Figure 11**).

In 2012, information on serogroup was reported for 3234 of confirmed IMD cases in EU countries including 68% of serogroup B, 17% of serogroup C (17%), and a total of 93% included B and C, Y [8]. It is clearly seen that in the EU and also in Ukraine IM case are due mostly to serogroup B, while serogroups B and C are less represented in Ukraine than in EU.

In 2008, serogroup C incidence of was 0.21 per 100,000 in Ukraine. In 2012, it dropped to 0.08 per 100,000. From 2008 to 2012, this index was slightly higher than the 0.1 per 100,000 in EU/EEA countries [9]. Thus, in the Ukraine, currently, the incidence of serogroup C is not different for EU/EEA but in Ukraine not carried out vaccination against Men C. This fact does not negate the benefits of vaccination but requires further detailed study. When one compares the incidence Men type C in EU with routine vaccination and Ukraine, where routine vaccination against MI has never been carried out, the effectiveness of Men C vaccination appears negligible because the incidence Men type C in EU and Ukraine is not different.

In Europe and Ukraine, decline in the incidence of other serogroups (A and B) was not the result of specific interventions. We believe that demographic situation in Ukraine population has decreased from 52 to 45 million over the past 25 years. Birth rate decreases, and therefore, child population falls, altogether this will certainly not contribute to an increase incidence of IMD in Ukraine for the coming decade. The introduction of routine vaccination of IMD in Ukraine requires careful study because there is limited funding for public health.

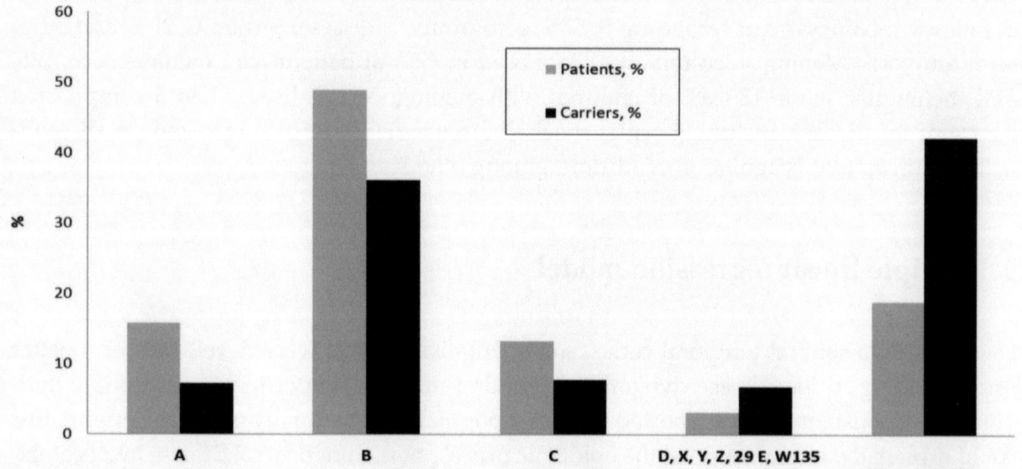

Figure 11. Distribution of meningococcus serogroups among patients with meningococcal disease (n = 9484) and healthy carriers of (n = 15,868), Ukraine, 1992–2012. Legend: Abscissa = Meningococcus serogroups; Ordinate = cases of meningococcal disease (%); red bar = healthy carriers of MI-pathogen (%); blue bar = patients with meningococcal disease (%).

4. Clinics

Among the 18,914 cases of IMD reported in Ukraine, 38.4% were meningococcemia, 29.9% were meningococcemia with meningitis, 27.9% meningitis and others 2.8% were of different minor etiologies. Other clinical forms have not been also clearly recognized and characterized as pneumonia or mixed clinical forms.

Also, the distribution of clinical forms of IMD in Ukraine is very different from the one observed in the EU countries in which meningitis prevails for 43.0%. Meningococcemia and meningococcemia with meningitis represent, respectively, 21.0 and 29.0% of total IMD in the EU [10].

Case fatality rate (CFR) of Meningococcal disease in Ukraine for the period considered (1992–2012) was of: 12.1% for IMD (n = 18,914); 18.9% for Meningococcemia (n = 7448); 10.1% for Meningococcemia (n = 5660); 5.94% of Meningitis (n = 5273); and 5.6% for others undefined clinical forms (n = 538).

In 2012, overall CFR in EU/EEA countries was 7.9%, (3185 confirmed IMD cases). The highest CFR reported (n = 1563) among cases presenting septicemia was 18.8%, followed by cases meningitis with septicemia of 11.1%, and then by cases with meningitis (3.7%) [11]. In Ukraine, the higher observed overall CFR of IMD greater than in the EU can be attributed to the frequency of septicemia.

Meningococcal disease CFR among children in Ukraine during the period of 2010–2015 ranged from 14.7 to 19.1% occurring as follows with respect to the age class: first year of life, 66%; 1–3-year old, 30%; over three-year old, 4%. Among 77% of patient death occurred during the first 24 h after onset.

According to the children's infectious hospital of Kiev, for the past 15 years, serotypes prevail as follows: meningococcal serogroup B, 57%; serogroup A, 19%; serogroup C, 20%; and other serogroup, 4%. Meningococcemia was diagnosed in 47% of patient with meningococcemia, 41% meningitis, while 12–76% of children with meningococcal disease had a complicated course of the disease, including septic shock, brain edema, multiple organ failure, disseminated intravascular coagulation syndrome, among others.

5. Multiple linear regression model

From this data set and temporal series, some tentative models were developed for a better understanding to the disease dynamics. Assuming that the proportion of susceptible individuals is a constant value a reported to a large population (eventually of genetic origin), this could explain the main feature of the epidemic process of meningococcal disease and ecological characteristics of meningococcus commensality.

Also, meningococcus as a species may exist as a non-pathogenic microorganism. IMD will then arise only among susceptible people who have a genetic predisposition while in any large population, such a percentage is very small (<1%).

In order to calculate the percentage of susceptible population to IMD, it is possible to calculate it as a risk of susceptibility (RS), the percentage of susceptible, i.e. approximate proportion of the population susceptible" (APPS) to IMD. In order to calculate APPS, we first calculate the annual estimated number of carriers, AAQC (infected people without clinical manifestations):

$$APPS = (IMD\ number{:}AAQC) \times 100\% \tag{1}$$

where AAQC = annual approximate quantity of carriers (infected people without clinical manifestations); CPR = carrier prevalence rate (from the ratio of the carriers detected among people examinees); N = the census of the population of the studied territory; 365 = days (i.e., a year); D = average duration of carriage status (not detected after 14 days).

where AAQC formula is derived from PR formula:

$$\mathrm{AAQC} = \frac{\mathrm{CPR} \times \mathrm{N} \times 365}{\mathrm{D}} \tag{2}$$

where PR = prevalence rate; IR = incidence rate; D = average day duration for one case of carriage [12].

Ultimately, AAQC formula allows to convert the data of sample surveys (i.e., prevalence of meningococcal carriage showed (**Figure 9**) to indicators of incidence (or the annual approximate number of carriers). Thus, we calculated the AAQC among healthy children for the period 1992–2012 years. The AAQC of children was calculated from 2,206,475 persons. The proportion of IMD cases (i.e., % susceptible) presented an average of 0.0360% ± 0.0189, that is: in overall, one IMD patient associated with 5271 carriers in during 1990–2012.

Moreover, this way we calculated indicators for period of time from 1992 to 2012 for the general population. The annual average number of carriers in the general healthy population was 24,990,502 persons (variation of 15,480,263–34,746,741 per year). The proportion of IMD cases (i.e., % susceptible) had an average of 0.0036% (0.0022–0.0058% per year), that is: one IMB patient associated an average of 29,729 carriers.

In overall, this is consistent with the fact that the IMD incidence among children exceeds IMD incidence in the general population (or adult) by 10-fold or more.

The total risk of disease (RD) is expressed as a product of risk of infection (RI) to risk of susceptibility (RS) where RD = RI × RS. Thus, in our paradigm, RS and RI are the final and necessary causes of IMD emergence and spread to human population. All other causes that may affect IMD incidence will act indirectly through RI and RS.

Therefore, we built multiple regression models of the epidemic process of MI, where the incidence of IMD is the dependent variable, while independent variables are the level of meningococcal carriage (RI) and the proportion of the susceptible population (RS). The construct of the regression model was by deriving multiple regression method [12]. Multiple linear regression models of IMD in Ukraine were therefore developed [13]. We used for the model the data presented in the figures 6 and 10.

Our first model takes the following form of the regression equation:

$$Y1 = -7.43 + 8.26\,X_1 + 227.63\,X_2, \tag{3}$$

where Y1 = IMD incidence per 100,000 children 0–14 years; −7.43 (or "a") = constant, which corresponds to the mathematical expectation X_1 and X_2 if Y = 0; X_1 = prevalence of carriage among healthy children aged 0–14 (%); X_2 = approximate proportion of the population susceptible to the IMD among children aged 0–14, or APPS (%); 8.26 (or "b_1") = regression coefficient showing the change of level Y, if X_1 is changed to 1%; 227.63 (or "b_2") = regression coefficient showing the change of level Y, if X_2 is changed to 1%.

Note that the influence of the regression coefficients (b_1 and b_2) and constant "a" at incidence Y is statistically significant (Student exact test: $b_1 = 14.56$ with $p = 2.13 \times 10^{-11}$; $b_2 = 15.39$ with $p = 8.38 \times 10^{-12}$; $a = 7.54$ with $p = 5.59 \times 10^{-7}$).

In the model, the coefficient of multiple correlation R = 0.9697 and its standard error is equal to 0.5069 ($R^2 = 0.9404$, i.e. 94.04%) that statistically significance explains IMD incidence and shows the high descriptive properties of the model. Ultimately, this model appears highly significant (Fisher's exact test = 142.04 $p < 0.05$ at 95% confidence) describing the totality of the properties of the epidemic process of MD among children aged 0–14. Analysis of the residuals values of the model did not find any autocorrelation. Overall, the model encompasses all properties and is statistically significant.

Our second model takes the following form of the regression equation:

$$Y2 = -1.59 + 0.89\,X_1 + 469.13\,X_2, \tag{4}$$

where Y2 = IMD incidence per 100,000 population; X_1 = prevalence of carriage among persons who had contact with IMD patients (or among total population), %; X_2 = approximate proportion of the population susceptible to the IMD among total population, APPSIMD, %. The model has excellent descriptive properties and statistically significant. The coefficient of multiple correlation r = 0.9937 and its standard error is equal to 0.0645, accordingly with r^2 = 0.9875. Residuals analysis of the model did not find any autocorrelation (i.e., almost normal distribution.)

Model limitation: Our models use aggregated data form a survey, and therefore, our model does not allow for an adequate formal residual analysis. In order to perform such type of analysis, it requires to build at least 50 times of such models from necessary data sets. Also, our models do not take into account the potential heterogeneity of the pathogen.

6. Conclusion

Altogether the present and past surveillance of bacterial meningitis in Ukraine provide a unique source for a comprehensive understanding of the disease dynamics and, most importantly, allow to develop tools and strategies for control and prevention.

Thus, the results of mathematical modeling of IMD using the available time series of data suggest that the nature of the main manifestations of the epidemic caused by the MI process demonstrates the prevalence of meningococcal carriage and provides a measure of the of susceptible populations, which are both factors strongly associated and allow the assessment of immediate risk of IMD in country. The proposed multiple linear regression model of epidemic process of meningococcal disease will improve epidemiological surveillance of the disease. Moreover, such models will provide a strong mean for assessing the quality of vaccination against invasive bacterial infections as well as diphtheria.

Acknowledgements

The authors would like to acknowledge the United States Department of Defense, Defense, Threat Reduction Agency (DTRA), Cooperative Biological Engagement Program (CBEP) for their support to develop this manuscript. While DTRA/CBEP did not support the research described in this publication, the Program supported the presentation of this research in an international forum and supported grantsmanship training related to the development of this manuscript. The contents of this publication are the responsibility of the authors and do not necessarily reflect the views of DTRA or the United States Government.

Author details

Hennadii Mokhort[1], Sergey Kramarev[1,2] and Jean-Paul J. Gonzalez[3]*

*Address all correspondence to: jpgonzalez@vet.k-state.edu

1 Bogomolets National Medical University, Kyiv, Ukraine

2 Ministry of Health of Ukraine, Kyiv, Ukraine

3 Kansas State University, Center of Excellence for Emerging Zoonosis and Animal Diseases CEEZAD, Manhattan KS, USA

References

[1] Jafri RZ, Ali A, Messonnier NE, et al. Global epidemiology of invasive meningococcal disease. Population Health Metrics. 2013;**11**:17. DOI: 10.1186/1478-7954-11-17

[2] WHO. Meningococcal Meningitis Fact Sheet N°141. Updated November, 2015

[3] Orr HJ, Gray SJ, Macdonald M, Stuart JM. Saliva and meningococcal transmission. Emerging Infectious Diseases. 2003;**9**:1314-1315

[4] Christensen H, May M, Bowen L, Hickman M, Trotter CL. Meningococcal carriage by age: A systematic review and meta-analysis. The Lancet Infectious Diseases. 2010;**10**(12):853-861

[5] The European Union Invasive Bacterial Infections Surveillance Network (EU-IBIS), 2006

[6] ECDC. European Centre for Disease Prevention and Control (ECDC). Annual Epidemiological Report Vaccine-preventable Diseases –Invasive Bacterial Diseases 2014. Stockholm: European Centre for Disease Prevention and Control (ECDC); 2014

[7] Mortality indicator database: Mortality indicators by 67 causes of death, age and sex (HFA-MDB), 2015. Available from: http://data.euro.who.int/hfamdb/tables/tableA.php?w=1024&h=768

[8] European Centre for Disease Prevention and Control (ECDC), 2015

[9] ECDC, 2015. Available from: http://ecdc.europa.eu/en/publications/Publications/Meningococcal-disease-scouts-EU-August-2015.pdf

[10] UNICEF, 2015. Available from: http://www.unicef.org/ukraine/about.html#Basic

[11] WHO, Control of epidemic meningococcal disease. WHO Practical Guidelines. 2nd ed. 1998

[12] Ahlbom A, Norell S. Introduction to Modern Epidemiology. Newton Lower Falls: Epidemiology Resources Inc. and New England Epidemiology Institute; 1990

[13] Glantz SA, Slinker BK. Primer of Applied Regression and Analysis of Variance. New York: McGraw–Hill; 1990

Chapter 3

Tick-Borne Encephalitis

Perta Bogovič and Franc Strle

Additional information is available at the end of the chapter

http://dx.doi.org/10.5772/intechopen.68366

Abstract

Tick-borne encephalitis (TBE) is an important central nervous system infection in Europe and Asia. It is caused by three subtypes of TBE virus (TBEV): European, Siberian and Far-Eastern, belonging to the genus *Flavivirus*. TBE is delineated by three criteria: the presence of clinical signs of meningitis, meningoencephalitis or meningoencephalomyelitis; cerebrospinal fluid pleocytosis ($>5 \times 10^6$ cells/L); and demonstration of a recent infection with TBEV by the presence of specific serum IgM and IgG antibodies or IgG seroconversion. Imaging of the brain and spinal cord has a low sensitivity and specificity, but it is useful for the differential diagnosis. Clinical course and outcome of TBE depend on the subtype of TBEV (the disease caused by the European subtype has a milder acute course and a more favorable long-term outcome than the disease caused by the other two virus subtypes), age of patients (increasing age is associated with more severe acute course and poorer outcome) and probably on some host genetic factors. Due to relatively severe clinical course combined with the absence of etiologic treatment, considerable proportion of patients with incomplete recovery after acute illness, and increasing incidence, TBE represents a growing (public) health problem that could be substantially reduced with vaccination.

Keywords: tick-borne encephalitis, tick-borne encephalitis virus, epidemiology, pathogenesis, clinical manifestations, diagnosis, treatment, prevention, vaccination

1. Introduction

Tick-borne encephalitis (TBE) is an important human viral infection of central nervous system (CNS) endemic in a large part of Europe and Asia. The causative agents are three different TBE virus (TBEV) subtypes named European, Siberian and Far-Eastern [1]. In spite of the pronounced genetic similarity of these flaviviruses, the illness caused by individual subtype is not entirely comparable to those caused by the other subtypes.

The clinical course of acute illness is highly variable. Due to the relatively high proportion of severe cases and a considerable proportion of patients with long-lasting sequelae which may have a significant impact on quality of life, the disease represents high costs for healthcare system and society.

Herein we present an overview of TBE, including a short historical outline, basic information on TBEV, and of the epidemiology, pathogenesis, clinical manifestations, diagnosis and treatment of TBE, as well as on the course and outcome of the disease and its prevention.

2. History

Historically the first mention of the TBE existence dates back to the eighteenth century in Scandinavian church records from Åland Islands. However, the first medical description of disease was given and published in 1931 by the Austrian physician H. Schneider [2]. Six years later, an expedition headed by Zilber in the Russian Far East isolated for the first time the causative agent (TBEV) from humans, mice, and *Ixodes persulcatus* ticks; they determined the etiology of TBE and its vector [3]. In 1939, Pavlovsky confirmed the preliminary hypothesis on the transmission of the TBEV in nature (between ticks and mammals) and proposed the theory of natural foci [4]. In Europe, TBEV was first isolated, from humans and *Ixodes ricinus* ticks, in Czechoslovakia in 1948 by Gallia and colleagues [5]. In the following years, the disease and/or the virus has been identified in many other European countries and, later, also in the north of China and northern Japan [6].

3. Etiology

TBE is caused by TBEV, a small, neurotropic, lipid-enveloped spherical RNA virus, the member of genus *Flavivirus*, family *Flaviviridae*. The viral RNA contains records for three structural (E (envelope), prM/M (precursor of membrane or membrane, respectively), and C (capsid)), and seven nonstructural viral proteins (NS1, NS2a, NS2b, NS3, NS4a, NS4b, and NS5). Glycoprotein E is a major viral antigen and is associated with the production of neutralizing antibodies and the induction of protective immunity. It also plays a key role in the viral life cycle mediating the binding of virions to cell receptors and subsequent intraendosomal fusion [7].

TBEV occurs in three subtypes named as European, Siberian, and Far-Eastern subtype [1]. They are very closely related, both genetically and antigenically; variation in amino acids sequences between subtypes is 5–6% [8]. In spite of the pronounced genetic similarity of the subtypes the illness caused by individual subtype is not completely equivalent to those due to the other subtypes.

An important characteristic of the TBEV, which allows them alimentary route of infection, is their ability to maintain at least residual infectivity at acidic pH (above pH 1.42) [9]. TBEV maintains infectivity at very low environment temperatures (even below −70°C). On the contrary, it is heat labile; total inactivation of the virus occurs within 30 minutes at 56°C [10, 11]. It can be inactivated by pasteurization [12].

http://dx.doi.org/10.5772/intechopen.68366

4. Epidemiology

TBE arises in an endemic pattern of so-called natural foci over a large geographical area extending from Central Europe and Scandinavia through the Eurasian continent to North-Eastern China and Northern Japan. Over the past few decades, a trend toward both an expansion of the endemic areas and an increase of reported cases have been observed [13, 14]. The increase in the incidence is the result of a complex interrelation of socioeconomic and ecological factors; a part of an increase may also be explained with an increased medical awareness, advanced diagnostics, and improvements in epidemiological surveillance [15, 16].

In Europe and Asia between 10,000 and 15,000 TBE cases are reported per year with pronounced annual fluctuations [17]. The number is very likely underreported mainly due to lack of standardized TBE case definition, the varying diagnostics procedures, and the wide differences in the quality of national surveillance systems.

In 2012, TBE became a notifiable disease at the European Union level. Currently the disease is endemic in 27 European countries; the reporting is mandatory in 18 of them. Two-thirds of the countries where TBE is a notifiable disease use the European Centre for Disease Prevention and Control case definition [13, 18, 19]. A total of 2560 TBE cases were reported in Europe in 2012 with the overall notification rate of 0.52 cases per 100,000 inhabitants. Countries with the highest reported incidence (>5 cases per 100,000 inhabitants per year) were Estonia (13.35), Lithuania (11.69), Slovenia (7.98), and Czech Republic (5.46) [20].

The main hosts and reservoirs of TBEV in nature are wild vertebrate, in particular small rodents. Ticks act as both virus vectors and reservoir and carry the virus throughout their life. Humans are only accidental hosts and do not play any role in the maintenance of TBEV in nature [21, 22].

Most human infections occur through an infected hard tick bites. At least 11 tick species are capable of transmitting TBEV, but only 2 species are of clinical importance. *I. ricinus* is the principal vector throughout Europe and, therefore, the most important transmitter of the European TBEV subtype, while *I. persulcatus* occurs in regions of Eastern Europe, in Russia, and in far-eastern Asia and is the main vector of the Siberian and Far-Eastern TBEV subtype [21, 23]. The Siberian TBEV subtype is found in Siberia, the Baltics, and northern Finland, whereas the Far-Eastern TBEV subtype is endemic in far-eastern Asia and Japan, and also in central and eastern Siberia [13, 22]. In the Baltic States and Finland, where *I. ricinus* overlaps with *I. persulcatus,* all three TBEV subtypes co-circulate [24–26]. The Far-Eastern TBEV was found in *Ixodes ovatus* in Japan in south-western China, while the European TBEV subtype was detected in *Ixodes nipponensis* ticks in Korea [1, 27].

In Europe, the TBEV prevalence in unfed *I. ricinus* ticks ranges from 0.1 to 5.0% (depending on the geographical location and time of the year) and increases with development stage, whereas in Siberia, the reported proportion of infected adult *I. persulcatus* ticks is up to 40% [13, 21]. In Slovenia, the prevalence of TBEV-infected ticks was found to be 0.47%; 0.54% in 2005 and 0.43% in 2006 [28]. About 1% of all human TBEV infections are alimentary-transmitted by consuming contaminated unpasteurized dairy products, especially goat milk [1]. This route of infection has to be considered in cases of local epidemics. The majority of outbreaks due to oral virus transmission are reported from Eastern Europe and Baltic states [29, 30]. A few cases of laboratory-acquired TBEV infections have been documented [31]. Vertical transmission, person-to-person transmission including breast-feeding, and transmission through blood transfusion have not been reliably described in humans.

TBE is a seasonal disease; most cases occur in the warm period of the year (usually between April and November) which correlates with the period of the highest tick activity and with increased exposure during this time period [32]. In Central Europe, a two-peak distribution of TBE cases can be seen, first in June and July, and second in September and October, whereas in the regions where *I. persulcatus* is widespread, cases as a rule occur in May and June [11]. In all age groups men are affected more frequently than women. The highest notification rate is in the 45–64 year-old age group, followed by the over 65-year olds [20, 33]. On an average, 10–20% of all reported cases of TBE occur in children, with the lowest incidence in those less than 3 years of age [34, 35]. It should be pointed out that due to its unspecific clinical presentation, TBE in children is often missed and is diagnosed as aseptic meningitis of unknown etiology [36, 37].

TBE represents a potential risk for nonvaccinated travelers traveling to countries with high endemic foci and therefore should be included in the differential diagnosis of the CNS infections in case of an appropriate epidemiological history also in patients living outside endemic areas. The risk depends on the season of travel, duration of stay as well as on travel style (degree of unprotected outdoor exposure). In the different endemic areas, the risk for infection after a single tick bite varies from 1:200 to 1:1000 [21].

5. Pathogenesis and pathology

After the bite of an infected tick TBEV replication occurs locally. Dendritic cells (Langerhans cells) are considered to be the most important cells for local viral replication and to transport the virus to the regional lymph nodes where further replication takes place. After release into the bloodstream the virus disseminate to other organs, in particular to the reticulo-endothelial system (mainly bone marrow, spleen, and liver) where the virus continue to multiply and maintain viremia for few days. During the viremic phase (which clinically matches to the initial phase of TBE) the virus probably reaches the brain [38, 39]. The precise mechanism of viral passage through the blood-brain barrier is unclear, but depends on the presence of viremia. Four possible routes have been postulated: (i) peripheral nerves, (ii) highly susceptible olfactory neurons (especially relevant in laboratory infections by aerosols), (iii) transcytosis through vascular endothelial cells of brain capillaries, and (iv) diffusion of the virus between capillary endothelial cells. The primary targets of TBEV infection in central nervous system are neurons. Rarely, oligodendrocytes are infected [38].

TBEV in CNS induces inflammation with inflammatory cell infiltration, activation of microglia, and neuronal degeneration. The exact mechanism of tissue destruction is unclear, but Ružek and coworkers demonstrated that inflammatory reaction mediated by CD8+ T cells significantly contributes to neuronal damage [40]. Limited data are available on the role of cytokines and chemokines.

Pathological lesions are widespread all over the CNS and involve leptomeninges and gray matter, with the brain stem, cerebellum, basal ganglia, thalamus, and spinal cord being most frequently affected. Histological findings are nonspecific; lesions consist of perivascular and parenchymal accumulation of lymphocytes, consisted of T and B cells, and macrophages (microglia), associated with nerve cells necrosis and neuronophagia in regions of viral replication. Residual lesions are characterized by loss of neurons and microglial scarring. Cerebral and spinal meninges usually show diffuse infiltration with lymphocytes and sometimes neutrophils. The most extensive meningeal inflammation is around the cerebellum [38, 41].

6. Clinical manifestations of TBEV infection

Seroepidemiological studies have demonstrated that TBEV infection is often asymptomatic. The exact proportion of such cases is not known, because those with mild clinical presentation may not be diagnosed, but data suggest rates between 70 and 98% [42–44].

Time interval from a tick bite to the beginning of the illness is usually 7–14 days, but it may be as short as 2 days and as long as 4 weeks. After alimentary route of infection, there is regularly a shorter incubation period of 3–4 days [30, 32, 45].

In at least three-quarters of patients who develop CNS involvement, the disease caused by the European virus subtype has a biphasic course [46–48]. The initial phase corresponds to the viremia and usually presents with nonspecific systemic signs and symptoms; the most common are moderate fever (99%), fatigue (63%), general malaise (62%), headache and body pain (arthralgia and myalgia) (54%) [47]. In this phase, which lasts 2–7 days, there are no signs or symptoms of CNS involvement; cerebrospinal fluid (CSF) examination reveals normal findings. After an improvement or even an asymptomatic interval of about 1 week duration (range 1–21 days) the second phase presents as meningitis, meningoencephalitis, or meningoencephalomyelitis in 54, 37, and 9% of adult patients [49]. The far most frequent clinical manifestation of TBE in children is meningitis [34]. Fever in the second phase is typically 1–2°C higher than the peek temperature in the first phase and is of longer duration [12, 50].

In some patients the disease course is monophasic: they may either have CNS involvement or a febrile illness with headache with symptoms subsiding without developing into the second phase (i.e., the initial phase of TBE without subsequent CNS involvement), named abortive form of TBE or "febrile headache" [12, 32, 50, 51].

6.1. Abortive form of TBE

Data on the frequency of this clinical manifestation of the disease caused by European TBEV subtype are conflicting. According to some reports it represents more than a half of all clinically manifested TBEV infections [32, 52]. However, this is not confirmed by the results of a prospective clinical trial on the etiology of acute febrile illness after a tick bite carried out by Lotric-Furlan and coworkers: of the 56 patients diagnosed with TBEV infection during the initial phase of illness, in 55 (98.2%), CNS involvement with pleocytosis later appeared, whereas only one (1.8%) had an isolated initial phase of the disease [51, 53]. In the Russian publications, this clinical manifestation is named "fever form" and is reported to represent up to 50% of all clinical presentations of TBE [54]. Abortive form of TBE most frequently presents itself by a moderate fever, headache, fatigue, and other nonspecific symptoms of the initial phase of the disease. The fever usually subsides in a few days and the disease does not have long-term consequences [55, 56].

6.2. Meningitis, encephalitis, and myelitis

Meningitis is characterized by fever, headache, nausea, vomiting, and meningeal signs. These symptoms and signs are present in the majority but not in all the patients. In a study encompassing 448 adult patients with TBE from Slovenia, almost all reported headache and had fever, more than 50% suffered from nausea and/or vomiting, and 70% had clearly expressed meningeal signs [33]. Encephalitis may manifest by a variety of neurological symptoms and signs, most often with tremor (especially of the fingers of the upper extremities and tongue), sometimes with nystagmus, speech disorder, ataxia and movement disorders, occasionally with seizures, and very rarely with brain stem symptoms and/or cranial nerve abnormalities. Impaired consciousness, ranging from mild to severe, insomnia, and concentration and cognitive function disturbances are rather frequent. Mental disorders including amnesia, behavioral changes, psychosis, and delirium may also occur. Patients may have sensory impairment. Myelitis is virtually always associated with meningoencephalitis, and as a rule manifests with flaccid paralyses that are occasionally preceded by severe pain in the affected muscle groups. The involvement is usually asymmetrical. Most often extremities are affected, more frequently the upper than the lower limbs, and more often the proximal segments of the extremities than the distal ones. Patients with pareses of respiratory muscles usually require artificial ventilatory support [12, 32, 57].

6.3. Other manifestations in the acute phase of illness

6.3.1. Involvement of cranial nerves

According to rather limited data, involvement of cranial nerves is rare, mostly asymmetrical, typically associated with severe acute illness, and usually has a favorable outcome [46, 47, 58]. Ocular, facial, and pharyngeal muscles are most often affected, but hearing and vestibular defects are also encountered [42].

In a series of 1218 adult patients diagnosed with TBE at a single center, 11 (0.9%) developed peripheral facial palsy (2 bilateral, 9 unilateral); however, 3 out of 11 patients had associated borrelial infection. The latter finding suggests that in patients who develop peripheral facial palsy in the course of TBE, and who had been exposed to ticks in the region where both TBE and Lyme borreliosis are endemic, coexistent infection with Lyme borreliae have to be taken into account [59].

6.3.2. Autonomic disorders

Occasionally, autonomic nervous system disorders are present in patients with TBE [60].

6.3.3. Encephalitis with normal CSF cell counts

Literature review revealed some reports on a serologically confirmed TBEV infection in patient with encephalitis but without CSF pleocytosis [61, 62]. This disagrees with the large series of serologically proven TBE patients, in which CSF pleocytosis was found in all the cases [12, 42, 43, 47]. However, the latter finding might be the result of a selection bias because in the studies CSF pleocytosis was one of the essential inclusion criteria for the diagnosis of TBE.

6.4. TBE in patients who had been vaccinated against the disease

It seems that breakthrough TBE after vaccination is rare: 7 cases were reported in Slovenia, 25 in Austria, and 27 in Sweden in the periods 2000–2006, 2000–2008, and 2002–2008, respectively. The majority (70%) of patients were over 50 years old, but also a pediatric case has been described [63–67]. According to Kunz, disease severity in unvaccinated and vaccinated patients with TBE does not differ substantially; however, the information is limited [68].

6.5. Chronic progressive TBE

A chronic progressive form of TBE, believed to be associated with the Siberian subtype of TBEV, has been described in Siberia and Far East. It may manifest with *epilepsia partialis continua* [69–72].

6.6. Postencephalitic syndrome

According to published data postencephalitic syndrome occurs in up to 58% of patients after acute TBE caused by European subtype of TBEV, and may include various nonspecific neurological/neuropsychiatric symptoms and residual neurological dysfunctions [73]. It often affects the patient's quality of life (sometimes requires a change in lifestyle) and also represents a high cost for the health care system and society.

The most commonly reported symptoms/signs have been cognitive or neuropsychiatric complaints (i.e., apathy, irritability, memory and concentration disorders, altered sleep pattern), headache, hearing defects, disturbances of vision, ataxia, and pareses or flaccid paralyses [46, 47, 58, 73, 74]. At this point it should be noted that most of the studies failed to include a control group; therefore, the findings are difficult to interpret due to unclear differences between postencephalitis syndrome, other consequences of TBE and symptoms present in the general population.

Lithuanian prospective clinical follow-up study showed that 46% of patients with TBE had sequelae 1 year post infection [47]. In 2009, Misić-Majerus et al. published a prospective study on TBE postencephalitic syndrome. One hundred and twenty-four patients, aged 16–76 years, participated in the study with follow-up period for at least 3 years. Forty-nine patients (39.5%) developed moderate or severe sequelae lasting for 3 to 18 months; in 11 patients permanent sequelae were seen—spinal nerve paresis in five, hearing impairment in six, dysarthria in two, and severe mental disorder in one patient [74]. In 2011, Kaiser reported 10-year follow-up results in patients with encephalomyelitic manifestation of TBE; 11 (19%) out of 57 included patients fully recovered, 29 (51%) patients had long-lasting sequelae (paresis or other impairments), and 17 (30%) died 1–10 years after the acute disease. The most substantial improvements were seen in the first year after acute disease [75]. Recently published case-control study on the long-term sequelae after TBE from Sweden has showed that the neurocognitive and motor symptoms in patients significantly differ from those in the age- and gender-matched control group [76].

7. Diagnosis

For a diagnosis of TBE, three criteria should be fulfilled:

(a) symptoms/signs indicating meningitis or meningoencephalitis,

(b) elevated CSF cell count (>5 × 10^6 leukocytes/L), and

(c) microbiologic evidence of TBEV infection (i.e., the presence of specific IgM and IgG antibodies) [77].

7.1. Blood and cerebrospinal fluid analysis

In the initial (viremic) phase of TBE leukopenia and/or thrombocytopenia are ascertained in around 70% of patients, and abnormal liver test results are seen in about 20% [78]. In the second (meningoencphalitic) phase, platelet count is normal, whereas peripheral blood leukocyte count is normal or mildly elevated (rarely >15 × 10^9/L). Concentration of C-reactive protein and erythrocyte sedimentation rate is usually in normal range throughout the entire course of TBE. In the initial phase of TBE, CSF findings are in the normal range, whereas in the second (meningoencephalitic) phase, elevated CSF leukocyte counts (usually <500 × 10^6/L, extremely rarely ≥1000 × 10^6/L), a normal to moderately elevated protein concentration, and a normal glucose concentration are present. A typical finding is lymphocytic pleocytosis; however, in the first few days of the meningoencephalitic phase of TBE, neutrophils may predominate in CSF. Elevated lymphocyte counts may persist for several weeks after clinical recovery [32, 79].

7.2. Magnetic resonance imaging (MRI) abnormalities

MRI abnormalities of brain and spinal cord are present only in about 20% of patients with TBE. According to a study performed by Kaiser [46], they are found more often in patients with meningoencephalomyelitis (7/25, 29%) than in patients with meningoencephalitis (11/64, 17%), and are not seen in those with meningitis (0/13). Increased signal intensity is most often seen in the thalamus, but can (also) be present in basal ganglia, internal capsule, splenium, cerebellum, peduncles and brain stem [46, 80–92]; in patients with myelitis, the abnormalities are seen predominantly in the anterior horns of the spinal cord [84, 85, 89, 93–97]. Studies of specificity are lacking but the specificity is probably low [89].

7.3. Microbiological investigations

7.3.1. Detection of TBEV

Due to limited diagnostic yield, direct approaches to demonstrate TBEV, such as detection of viral RNA by reverse transcriptase PCR and isolation of the virus, are as a rule not used in clinical practice. TBEV is present in blood in the initial (viremic) phase of TBE but not in the meningoencephalitic phase of the disease and is only very exceptionally present in CSF [98].

7.3.2. Serology

In the routine clinical practice, demonstration of antibodies to TBEV in serum (and in some cases also in CSF) by enzyme-linked immunosorbent assay (ELISA) is a standard microbiologic diagnostic approach with a high sensitivity and specificity [98, 99]. At the beginning of the meningoencephalitic phase, when patients are usually seen by their physicians and admitted to hospital, the large majority had specific serum IgM and IgG antibodies. In rare cases when only IgM antibodies to TBEV are found in the first serum sample, second sampling 1–2 weeks later reveals IgG seroconversion and enables a reliable diagnosis of (recent) TBEV infection. In CSF, IgM and IgG antibodies to TBEV appear several days later than in serum, but are detectable in almost all cases by day 10 [98, 100].

Although the interpretation of the results of serological testing is usually straightforward, there may be some obstacles which should be taken into account. TBEV IgM antibodies may be present in serum for several months (up to 10 months or even longer) after acute infection, whereas TBEV IgG antibodies persist for a whole life and mediate an immunity that prevents symptomatic reinfection [98, 101].

Thus, serum IgG antibodies to TBEV without the presence of specific IgM antibodies do not indicate a recent but previous (symptomatic or asymptomatic) TBEV infection or vaccination against TBE. On the other hand, specific TBE serum IgM antibodies, an indicator of a recent infection with TBEV, may be detectable for several months after acute TBEV infection (and also in some persons after the first two doses of primary immunization); their demonstration may result in incorrect interpretation if another CNS infection/disease developed within this time period [98, 101].

A further challenge is a close antigenic relationship between TBEV and other flaviviruses with cross-reactive antibodies induced by infections or vaccinations, and a consequent diagnostic difficulties in persons vaccinated against Japanese encephalitis or yellow fever and in travelers having acquired dengue, West Nile or other flavivirus infections [7]. Such problems in TBE serodiagnosis can be sorted out by the quantification of IgM antibodies. High IgM values (>500 arbitrary units) are indicative of a recent infection with TBEV, whereas lower IgM levels may require the analysis of a follow-up sample (that enables the assessment of antibody dynamics), and/or a specific neutralization assay, to rule out cross-reactive IgM antibodies and prolonged persistence of IgM antibodies after infection or vaccination [102].

Knowledge in the understanding of TBE serology is required also in patients with meningitis or meningoencephalitis or who had been previously vaccinated against TBE. Serological response in patients with TBE vaccination breakthroughs is as a rule distinct from the response in patients who had not been vaccinated; unawareness of the pattern may result in fail to notice vaccination breakthrough cases. Serologic response in these patients is characterized by a delayed development of specific IgM response (during the initial days of the meningoencephalitic phase of TBE, specific IgM antibodies may not be detectable) associated with a high and rapidly increasing levels of specific serum IgG antibodies [63, 64, 67]. For a reliable diagnosis of TBE in persons previously vaccinated against TBE, demonstration of intrathecal production of TBEV antibodies is needed [45].

8. Factors influencing clinical course of acute disease and/or long-term outcome

8.1. Subtype of TBEV

Subtype of TBEV influences the course of acute TBE as well as its long-term outcome. The disease caused by the European TBEV subtype usually has a biphasic course, around 10% of adult patients have a severe neurologic deficit, case-fatality rate is <2% [12, 32]. According to a prospective study the abortive form of TBE is rare—the initial phase most of the time move on to the second phase of the disease [51]. Long-lasting sequelae are identified in up to 50% of adult patients [103]. The disease is less severe and has a better outcome in children than in adults [34, 50, 104, 105].

Symptomatic infections with Far Eastern TBEV subtype often cause an illness with a gradual onset, more severe course, higher rates of severe neurologic sequelae, and a fatality rate of 20–40%; the severity and outcome in adults and children are similar. Limited information about the clinical course of the disease is available for Siberian TBEV subtype. The case-fatality rate is 2–3%; some reports from Russia suggest an association with a chronic progressive form of TBE [1, 11].

8.2. Age of patients

Published data suggest the relationship between age of patients and the severity of TBE and its outcome — the severity of acute illness and the proportion of patients with unfavorable outcome increase with age [33, 47, 50, 106].

The disease caused by European subtype of TBEV generally has a milder course and better outcome in children than in adults. The predominant form of TBE in children and adolescents is meningitis. A summary of 8 studies on 1169 children with TBE showed that meningitis was present in 802 (69%), meningoencephalitis in 356 (30%), and meningoencephalomyelitis in 11 (1%) patients. A total of 20 out of 945 patients (2.1%) had long-term neurologic sequelae [34]. In contrary to children, in adults, and especially in elderly patients with TBE caused by European subtype of TBEV, the most frequent presentation is meningoencephalitis [33, 47].

Furthermore, fatality rate, the ratio of patients who develop pareses, and the frequency of postencephalic syndrome is also parallel with the increasing age [33, 47, 106].

8.3. Other factors associated with severe acute disease

Some clinical studies have shown that TBE with monophasic presentation is associated with a more severe course of the acute disease [42, 107–111].

Concomitant TBE and Lyme neuroborreliosis may occur with a more severe clinical course [59, 112, 113].

8.4. Severity of acute illness and other risk factors for unfavorable outcome

The outcome of TBE is associated with clinical presentation. The risk of incomplete recovery is higher for patients who have more severe clinical illness during acute phase of TBE [45, 47].

Other identified risk factors found to be associated with unfavorable outcome are CSF cell count > 300 cells/μL, impaired blood-brain barrier (total protein >600 mg/L) and abnormal findings on MRI [46].

8.5. Genetic factors

Host-related factors, particularly genetically determined variability of the inflammatory/immune response, very likely have an important impact on the course and long-term outcome of TBE. In 2008, Kindberg and coworkers published the results of the study carried out on the Lithuanians, showing that a mutation in a chemokine receptor 5 (CCR5) gene increases the risk for the development of TBE after TBEV infection, but not for more severe disease [114]. Three years later the same group reported on an association between the wild-type Toll-like receptor 3 (TLR3) rs3775291 allele and increased risk of TBE and suggested that a functional TLR3 may be associated with disease severity [115]. Similar findings were also reported by Mickiene et al. [116]. Furthermore, Barkhash and coworkers found an association between polymorphism in the promoter region of CD209 gene and predisposition to severe illness, and a possible association between 5 OAS single nucleotide polymorphisms and the TBEV infection outcome in Russians [117, 118].

In the future we expect new interesting discoveries on the role of host genetic factors in TBEV infections.

9. Differential diagnosis

In addition to a variety of viral infections, differential diagnosis of the initial (viremic) phase of TBE includes also several diseases caused by bacteria. There is a striking similarity in clinical and laboratory presentation of the initial phase of TBE and human granulocytic anaplasmosis. For both diseases fever, headache, leukopenia, and thrombocytopenia are typical. However, the presence of clinical symptoms such as chills, myalgia and arthralgia, and laboratory findings of elevated concentration of C-reactive protein and lactate dehydrogenase values direct toward the diagnosis of human granulocytic anaplasmosis and against the initial phase of TBE [119].

TBE needs to be differentiated from encephalitis or aseptic meningitis due to many other viruses. Differential diagnosis comprises also other tick-borne diseases such as Lyme borreliosis, babesiosis, human granulocytic anaplasmosis, tick-transmitted rickettsioses, and tularemia. Since these diseases are treatable with antibiotics, caution must be taken to distinguish them from TBE [32].

Concomitant TBEV and *Borrelia burgdorferi* sensu lato infections, as well as concomitant TBEV and *Anaplasma phagocytophilum* infections have been described [77, 113, 120–122].

10. Treatment

There is no specific antiviral treatment for TBE. Patients as a rule need hospitalization, supportive care, symptomatic treatment based on the presence and severity of signs/symptoms and therapy of neurologic and systemic complications. The symptomatic treatment usually includes antipyretics, analgesics, antiemetics, maintenance of fluid and electrolyte balance, and if necessary administration of anticonvulsive agents and treatment of cerebral edema [50, 123–125].

In some countries corticosteroids are often used in patients with TBE. However, until reliable studies prove the benefits of corticosteroids, their usage for the treatment of TBE is not recommended [47, 126].

Several patients need intensive care management; in those with neuromuscular paralysis leading to respiratory failure, intubation and ventilatory support are required. In a large prospective study, encompassing 635 patients diagnosed with TBE in the period from 1994 to 1998 in Germany, 12% of patients were treated in intensive care unit and 5% of patients required assisted ventilation [46]. Among patients with TBE, treated at a single medical center in Slovenia in the period from 2000 to 2004, 6.9% were hospitalized in the intensive care unit and 22.5% of them needed mechanical ventilation [33].

11. Prevention

11.1. Nonspecific preventive measures

TBEV is transmitted to humans by a tick bite or consumption of infected milk. Therefore, nonspecific preventive measures consist of reduction of tick population, personal protective procedures, and—as milk from endemic regions may contain TBEV—pasteurization of milk, and avoiding consumption of unpasteurized milk and dairy products [30, 42].

Tick population can be diminished by taking environmental measures, such as control of deer population, treatment with acaricides, and/or regular cutting of grass around the residence.

Nonspecific personal preventive measures include avoidance of ticks (i.e. avoidance of contact with vegetation, especially in deciduous and mixed forests with a rich understory), wearing light-colored clothing (light colors enable that ticks are better noticeable) with long sleeves and slacks stuck in socks or footwear (to diminish tick access to the skin), use of repellents, careful examination of the whole body for the presence of ticks, and removal of the attached ticks as soon as possible. However, TBEV is present in salivary glands of the infected tick and may be transmitted from the saliva within a few minutes after attachment [42]. Although the recommended personal measures for the prevention of tick-borne diseases such as TBE and Lyme borreliosis appear to be obvious, the efficiency of some of these procedures is inadequate, uncertain or has not been properly evaluated. Furthermore, in everyday life only a small proportion of exposed persons follow the recommended procedures [127, 128].

11.2. Prevention with immunoglobulins (passive immunization)

In the TBE endemic regions, immunoglobulins containing gamma globulin against TBEV had been used as postexposure prophylaxis within 96 hours after a tick bite. Because protection was rather unreliable [129], and because several reports pointed toward a more severe disease course in children who had received the immunoglobulin [81, 129, 130], passive immunization (the usage of the immunoglobulins) in the European Union has been abandoned [131]. However, the specific immunoglobulins are still used in Russia; the reported protection rate is about 80% [132].

11.3. Vaccination

Active immunization is the most effective and reliable way to prevent TBE [12, 42].

11.3.1. Recommendations for TBE vaccination

Given that TBE occurrence varies within and between individual endemic areas, vaccination strategies need to incorporate risk assessments for a particular region. According to WHO recommendations [133], in highly endemic TBE regions (≥5 cases/100,000/year) vaccination should be offered to whole population, including children, whereas in regions with a moderate or low TBE incidence (<5 cases/100,000/year), immunization has to target individuals at risk, i.e., those having outdoor activities or working under high-risk conditions. Travelers from non-endemic to endemic areas should be vaccinated if extensive outdoor activities are expected [133–136].

Similarly, Central European Vaccination Awareness Group (CEVAG) strongly recommends the introduction of universal TBE vaccination for persons >1-year old for all countries at high risk of TBE [135]. Persons who had acquired TBE do not need vaccination as they are appreciated to be protected against the disease.

11.3.2. Vaccines

In Europe two vaccines against TBE are registered: FSME-IMMUN® and Encepur® (in some countries named TicoVac). Both contain inactivated European subtype of TBEV (strain Neudorf

1 and strain K23, respectively), are prepared in a similar way (viruses are grown in chick embryo fibroblast cells, are inactivated by formaldehyde and are purified, adjuvant is aluminum hydroxide), are registered for adults and children aged 1 year and older (vaccines for children are called FSME-IMMUN 0.25 ml Junior, and Encepur Kinder, respectively), and effectively prevent TBE caused by the European as well as Far-Eastern and Siberian subtype of TBEV [131].

In addition to the European vaccines, three vaccines based on Far-Eastern subtype of TBEV are registered: two are produced in Russia (TBE-Moscow and EnceVir) and one in China [131].

11.3.3. Vaccination schedule

All of several vaccination schedules consist of primary (basic) vaccination followed by booster doses. Complete primary (basic) vaccination comprises three doses, usually given with an interval of 1–3 months between first and second dose, and 5–12 months between the second and third dose. When protection is wanted to be achieved in a short time, "fast schedule" (second dose is administered earlier, usually 14 days instead of 1–3 months after the first dose) can be used in accordance with the manufacturers' instructions [12, 42]. The first booster dose is administered 3 years after completion of the primary vaccination; after that, one dose is required every 5 years except for persons aged >60 years (FSME IMMUN) or >50 years (Encepur) for whom boosters are recommended at 3 years intervals [131]. Immunization with the first two doses is preferably accomplished during the winter months to achieve protection before tick activity; however, vaccination can start at any time. A person who had not received the recommended doses according to the schedule but with longer intervals does not need to start vaccination again from the very beginning but just to continue with missing doses. Longer intervals between doses generally do not reduce antibody concentrations after completion of TBE vaccination, but protection in the period before the delayed dose is less consistent [137].

11.3.4. Mode of application and dosages

TBE vaccine is administered intramuscularly into the deltoid muscle; in young children, it can be given in the muscles of anterolateral thigh. It may be administered simultaneously with other vaccines (live or inactivated) but not on the same place [131]. Doses (0.25 or 0.5 ml) depend upon the age of the recipient. The age limits for vaccines available in Europe differ. In persons <16 years old, the dose of the FSME-IMMUN vaccine is 0.25 ml, whereas for persons ≥16 years, 0.5 ml is advised; the corresponding age limits for Encepur vaccine are <12 and ≥12 years, respectively.

11.3.5. Efficacy and safety

Both European vaccines are safe and effective. Fourteen days after the second dose of basic vaccination protective antibodies develop in about 85% of the subjects, whereas after three doses, more than 98% of persons with normal immunity are protected [131]. As a rule the effectiveness of protection after vaccination against TBE is not verified by the detection of antibodies against TBEV in serum. However, the manufacturers of the vaccines and some authors recommend that in persons with immunodeficiency, the response to vaccination is assessed by serological testing approximately 4 weeks after the second dose, and that — if

http://dx.doi.org/10.5772/intechopen.68366

antibody response was not adequate — the second dose is repeated and followed by the third dose in accordance with the regular TBE vaccination timetable. Along with some proposals similar procedure may possibly refer also to the following doses. While such practice may appear reasonable, no convincing clinical data corroborate its usage.

TBE vaccine field effectiveness is estimated to be >98% in persons vaccinated in line with the advocated schedule, and >90% for those who received basic vaccination, but were later not vaccinated according to the planned timetable [138].

Side effects are mild and relatively rare. They are more frequent after the initial than with later doses of TBE vaccine. The most common side effects are local pain and tenderness on pressure at the injection site; redness and swelling occur less often. Short-term fever after vaccination is relatively common in young children but rare in adults. Neurological complications are very infrequent [131].

11.3.6. Contraindications and limitations

11.3.6.1. Contraindications

The main contraindications are as follows:

a. Severe allergic reaction following preceding dose of TBE vaccine;

b. Information on severe allergic reactions to vaccine constituents (in addition to the active ingredients, TBE vaccine also contains remains of formaldehyde, protamine sulfate, gentamicin and neomycin); and

c. History on anaphylactic hypersensitivity to eggs (TBE viruses are grown in fibroblast cells of chick embryo).

d. Vaccination is not performed in persons with acute febrile illness.

11.3.6.2. Limitations

Pregnancy, breast-feeding: Because information on the safety of TBE vaccine during pregnancy and lactation is inadequate, pregnant and lactating women should receive the vaccine only after a careful individual assessment of the potential risks and benefits. There is also no sufficient data on the safety of vaccination during lactation. However, since TBE vaccines are based on inactivated virus, the harm of breast-feeding child or fetus is unlikely.

Autoimmune diseases: While there is no indication that vaccination may deteriorate the course of autoimmune diseases or trigger autoimmunity, caution is required in persons with an autoimmune disease because data on the safety of vaccination in this group are limited [131].

11.3.7. Storage

The vaccine must be stored in a refrigerator at a temperature between 2 and 8°C. Storage at higher temperatures and freezing are not suitable [131].

12. Conclusion

TBE is an important central nervous system infection endemic in European and Asian countries. Due to relatively high proportion of cases with severe clinical course and a considerable proportion of patients with permanent sequelae after acute illness, as well as due to high incidence, it represents a growing (public) health problem that could be substantially reduced with vaccination.

Author details

Perta Bogovič and Franc Strle*

*Address all correspondence to: franc.strle@kclj.si

Department of Infectious Diseases, University Medical Centre Ljubljana, Ljubljana, Slovenia

References

[1] Mansfield KL, Johnson N, Phipps LP, Stephenson JR, Fooks AR, Solomon T. Tick-borne encephalitis virus – A review of an emerging zoonosis. Journal of General Virology. 2009;**90**:1781-1794. DOI: 10.1099/vir.0.011437-0

[2] Schneider H. Über epidemische acute meningitis serosa. Wiener Klinische Wochenschrift. 1931;**44**:350-352

[3] Zilber LA. Spring-summer tick-borne encephalitis (in Russian). Arkhiv Biologicheskikh Nauk. 1939;**56**:255-261

[4] Pavlovsky EN. Ticks and tick-borne encephalitis (in Russian). Parazitologia Dalnego Vostoka Leningrad. 1947;**5**:212-264

[5] Gallia F, Rampas J, Hollender J. Laboratori infekce encefalitickym virem (in Czech). Casopis Lékaru Ceských. 1949;**88**:224-229

[6] Kunz C, Heinz FX. Tick-borne encephalitis. Vaccine. 2003;**21**(**Suppl** 1):S1–S2

[7] Heinz FX, Stasny K. Flaviviruses and their antigenic structure. Journal of Clinical Virology. 2012;**55**:289-295. DOI: 10.1016/j.jcv.2012.08.024

[8] Ecker M, Allison SL, Meixner T, Heinz FX. Sequence analysis and genetic classification of tick-borne encephalitis viruses from Europe and Asia. Journal of General Virology. 1999;**80**:179-185. DOI: 10.1099/0022-1317-80-1-179

[9] Stiasny K, Allison SL, Mandl CW, Heinz FX. Role of metastability and acidic pH in membrane fusion by tick-borne encephalitis virus. Journal of Virology. 2001;**75**:7392-7398. DOI: 10.1128/JVI.75.16.7392-7398.2001

[10] Gould EA. Virus cryopreservation and storage. Methods in Molecular Biology. 1995; **38**:7-20. DOI: 10.1385/0-89603-296-5:7

[11] Gritsun TS, Lashkevich VA, Gould EA. Tick-borne encephalitis. Antiviral Research. 2003;**57**:129-146

[12] Kaiser R. Tick-borne encephalitis. Infectious Disease Clinics of North America. 2008;**22**: 561-575. DOI: 10.1016/j.idc.2008.03.013

[13] Süss J. Tick-borne encephalitis 2010: Epidemiology, risk areas, and virus strains in Europe and Asia – An overview. Ticks and Tick-Borne Diseases. 2011;**2**:2-15. DOI: 10.1016/j.ttbdis.2010.10.007

[14] Amicizia D, Domnich A, Panatto D, Lai PL, Cristina ML, Avio U, Gasparini R. Epidemiology of tick-borne encephalitis (TBE) in Europe and its prevention by available vaccines. Human Vaccines & Immunotherapeutics. 2013;**9**:1163-1171. DOI: 10.4161/hv.23802

[15] Randolph SE. EDEN-TBD sub-project team. Human activities predominate in determining changing incidence of tick-borne encephalitis in Europe. Euro Surveillance. 2010;**15**:24-31

[16] Süss J. Tick-borne encephalitis in Europe and beyond – The epidemiological situation as of 2007. Euro Surveillance. 2008;**13**:18916

[17] Dobler G. Zoonotic tick-borne flaviviruses. Veterinary Microbiology. 2010;**140**:221-228. DOI: 10.1016/j.vetmic.2009.08.024

[18] European Centre for Disease Prevention and Control. ECDC Technical Report. Epidemiological Situation of Tick-Borne Encephalitis in the European Union and European Free Trade Association countries [Internet]. 2012. Available from: http://ecdc.europa.eu/en/publications/publications/tbe-in-eu-efta.pdf [Accessed: August 10, 2016]

[19] Amato-Gauci A, Zeller H. Tick-borne encephalitis joins the diseases under surveillance in the European Union. Euro Surveillance. 2012;**17**:20299

[20] European Centre for Disease Prevention and Control. ECDC Surveillance Report. Annual Epidemiological Report, Emerging and Vector-Borne Diseases, 2014 [Internet]. 2014. Available from: http://ecdc.europa.eu/en/publications/publications/emerging-vector-borne-diseases_annual-epidemiological-report-2014.pdf [Accessed: August 10, 2016]

[21] Süss J. Epidemiology and ecology of TBE relevant to the production of effective vaccines. Vaccine. 2003;**21**(Suppl 1):S19–S35

[22] Dobler G, Gniel D, Petermann R, Pfeffer M. Epidemiology and distribution of tick-borne encephalitis. Wiener Medizinische Wochenschrift Wiener Medizinische Wochenschrift. 2012;**162**:230-238. DOI: 10.1007/s10354-012-0100-5

[23] Kollaritsch H, Krasilnikov V, Holzmann H, Karganova G, Barre A, Süss J, Pervikov Y, Bjorvatn B, Duclos P, Hombach J. Background Document on Vaccines and Vaccination Against Tick-Borne Encephalitis (TBE) [Internet]. 2011. Available from: http://www.who.int/immunization/sage/6_TBE_backgr_18_Mar_net_apr_2011.pdf [Accessed: August 15, 2016]

[24] Lundkvist K, Vene S, Golovljova I, Mavtchoutko V, Forsgren M, Kalnina V, Plyusnin A. Characterization of tick-borne encephalitis virus from Latvia: Evidence for co-circulation of three distinct subtypes. Journal of Medical Virology. 2001;**65**:730-735

[25] Golovljova I, Vene S, Sjölander KB, Vasilenko V, Plyusnin A, Lundkvist A. Characterization of tick-borne encephalitis virus from Estonia. Journal of Medical Virology. 2004;**74**:580-588. DOI: 10.1002/jmv.20224

[26] Jääskeläinen AE, Tikkakoski T, Uzcátegui NY, Alekseev AN, Vaheri A, Vapalahti O. Siberian subtype tick-borne encephalitis virus, Finland. Emerging Infectious Diseases. 2006;**12**:1568-1571. DOI: 10.3201/eid1210.060320

[27] Kim SY, Yun SM, Han MG, Lee IY, Lee NY, Jeong YE, Lee BC, Ju YR. Isolation of tick-borne encephalitis viruses from wild rodents, South Korea. Vector-Borne and Zoonotic Diseases. 2008;**8**:7-13. DOI: 10.1089/vbz.2006.0634

[28] Durmiši E, Knap N, Saksida A, Trilar T, Duh D, Avšič-Županc T. Prevalence and molecular characterization of tick-borne encephalitis virus in Ixodes ricinus ticks collected in Slovenia. Vector-Borne and Zoonotic Diseases. 2011;**11**:659-664. DOI: 10.1089/vbz.2010.0054

[29] Křiz B, Benes C, Daniel M. Alimentary transmission of tick-borne encephalitis in the Czech Republic (1997-2008). Epidemiology Microbiology Immunology. 2009;**58**:98-103

[30] Hudopisk N, Korva M, Janet E, Simetinger M, Grgič-Vitek M, Gubenšek J, Natek V, Kraigher A, Strle F, Avšič-Županc T. Tick-borne encephalitis associated with consumption of raw goat milk, Slovenia, 2012. Emerging Infectious Diseases. 2013;**19**:806-808. DOI: 10.3201/eid1905.121442

[31] Avsic-Zupanc T, Poljak M, Maticic M, Radsel-Medvescek A, LeDuc JW, Stiasny K, Kunz C, Heinz FX. Laboratory acquired tick-borne meningoencephalitis: Characterisation of virus strains. Clinical and Diagnostic Virology. 1995;**4**:51-59

[32] Dumpis U, Crook D, Oksi J. Tick-borne encephalitis. Clinical Infectious Diseases. 1999;**28**: 882-890. DOI: 10.1086/515195

[33] Logar M, Bogovic P, Cerar D, Avsic-Zupanc T, Strle F. Tick-borne encephalitis in Slovenia from 2000 to 2004: Comparison of the course in adult and elderly patients. Wiener klinische Wochenschrift. 2006;**118**:702-707. DOI: 10.1007/s00508-006-0699-6

[34] Arnez M, Avsic-Zpanc T. Tick-borne encephalitis in children: An update on epidemiology and diagnosis. Expert Review of Anti-infective Therapy. 2009;**7**:1251-1260. DOI: 10.1586/eri.09.99

[35] Kunze U, Asokliene L, Bektimirov T, Busse A, Chmelik V, Heinz FX, Hingst V, Kadar F, Kaiser R, Kimmig P, Kraigher A, Krech T, Linquist L, Lucenko I, Rosenfeldt V, Ruscio M, Sandell B, Salzer H, Strle F, Süss J, Zilmer K, Mutz I. Tick-borne encephalitis in childhood – Consensus 2004. Wiener Medizinische Wochenschrift. 2004;**154**:242-245

[36] Hansson ME, Orvell C, Engman ML, Wide K, Lindquist L, Lidefelt KJ, Sundin M. Tick-borne encephalitis in childhood: Rare or missed? The Pediatric Infectious Disease Journal. 2011;**30**:355-357. DOI: 10.1097/INF.0b013e3181fe3b5a

[37] Sundin M, Hansson ME, Engman ML, Orvell C, Lindquist L, Wide K, Lidefelt KJ. Pediatric tick-borne infections of the central nervous system in an endemic region of Sweden: A prospective evaluation of clinical manifestations. European Journal of Pediatrics. 2012;**171**:347-352. DOI: 10.1007/s00431-011-1542-2

[38] Ružek D, Dobler G, Donoso Mantke O. Tick-borne encephalitis: Pathogenesis and clinical implications. Travel Medicine and Infectious Disease. 2010;**8**:223-232. DOI: 10.1016/j.tmaid.2010.06.004

[39] Mandl CW. Steps of the tick-borne encephalitis virus replication cycle that affect neuropathogenesis. Virus Research. 2005;**111**:161-174. DOI: 10.1016/j.virusres.2005.04.007

[40] Ruzek D, Salát J, Palus M, Gritsun TS, Gould EA, Dyková I, Skallová A, Jelínek J, Kopecký J, Grubhoffer L. CD8+ T-cells mediate immunopathology in tick-borne encephalitis. Virology. 2009;**384**:1-6. DOI: 10.1016/j.virol.2008.11.023

[41] Gelpi E, Preusser M, Laggner U, Garzuly F, Holzmann H, Heinz FX, Budka H. Inflammatory response in human tick-borne encephalitis: Analysis of postmortem brain tissue. Journal of Neurovirology. 2006;**12**:322-327. DOI: 10.1080/13550280600848746

[42] Lindquist L, Vapalahti O. Tick-borne encephalitis. Lancet. 2008;**371**:1861-1871. DOI: 10.1016/S0140-6736(08)60800-4

[43] Gustafson R, Svenungsson B, Forsgren M, Gardulf A, Granström M. Two-year survey of the incidence of Lyme borreliosis and tick-borne encephalitis in a high-risk population in Sweden. European Journal of Clinical Microbiology Infectious Diseases. 1992;**11**:894-900

[44] Libikova H. Epidemiological and clinical aspects of tick-borne encephalitis in reaction to multiple viral infections. In: Proceedings of Tick-Borne Encephalitis, an International Symposium (Baden). Vienna: Facultas Verlag; 1981. pp. 235-246

[45] Bogovic P, Strle F. Tick-borne encephalitis: A review of epidemiology, clinical characteristics, and management. World Journal of Clinical Cases. 2015;**3**:430-441. DOI: 10.12998/wjcc.v3.i5.430

[46] Kaiser R. The clinical and epidemiological profile of tick-borne encephalitis in southern Germany 1994-98: A prospective study of 656 patients. Brain. 1999;**122**:2067-2078

[47] Mickiene A, Laiskonis A, Günther G, Vene S, Lundkvist A, Lindquist L. Tick-borne encephalitis in an area of high endemicity in Lithuania: Disease severity and long-term prognosis. Clinical Infectious Diseases. 2002;**35**:650-658. DOI: 10.1086/342059

[48] Günther G, Haglund M, Lindquist L, Forsgren M, Sköldenberg B. Tick-bone encephalitis in Sweden in relation to aseptic meningoencephalitis of other etiology: A prospective study of clinical course and outcome. Journal of Neurology. 1997;**244**:230-238

[49] Kaiser R. Clinical Description. Tick-Borne Encephalitis (TBE, FSME) [Internet]. 2007. Available from: http://www.tbe-info.com/upload/medialibrary/Monograph_TBE.pdf [Accessed: August 15, 2016].

[50] Bogovic P, Lotric-Furlan S, Strle F. What tick-borne encephalitis may look like: Clinical signs and symptoms. Travel Medicine and Infectious Disease. 2010;**8**:246-250. DOI: 10.1016/j.tmaid.2010.05.011

[51] Lotrič-Furlan S, Avšič-Županc T, Strle F. An abortive form of tick-borne encephalitis (TBE) – A rare clinical manifestation of infection with TBE virus. Wiener Klinische Wochenschrift. 2002;**114**:627-629

[52] Kunz C. Tick-borne encephalitis in Europe. Acta Leidensia. 1992;**60**:1-14

[53] Lotric-Furlan S, Avsic-Zupanc T, Strle F. Is an isolated initial phase of a tick-borne encephalitis a common event? Clinical Infectious Diseases. 2000;30:987-988. DOI: 10.1086/313838

[54] Ustinova OU, Volechova GM, Devitkov MI, Gusmanova AI. The clinico-epidemiological characteristics of tick-borne encephalitis in the Perm Province (in Russian). Zhurnal Mikrobiologii Epidemiologii Immunobiologii. 1997;**3**:33-36

[55] Misić-Majerus L, Bujić N, Madarić V, Avsic-Zupanc T. An abortive type of tick-borne meningoencephalitis (in Croatian). Acta Medica Croatica. 2003;**57**:111-116

[56] Meyer PM, Zimmermann H, Goetschel P. Tick-borne encephalitis presenting as fever without localising signs – A case series. European Journal of Pediatrics. 2010;**169**:767-769. DOI: 10.1007/s00431-009-1097-7

[57] Fauser S, Stich O, Rauer S. Unusual case of tick-borne encephalitis with isolated myeloradiculitis. Journal of Neurology, Neurosurgery, and Psychiatry. 2007;**78**:909-910. DOI: 10.1136/jnnp.2006.110882

[58] Haglund M, Forsgren M, Lindh G, Lindquist L. A 10-year follow-up study of tick-borne encephalitis in the Stockholm area and a review of the literature: Need for a vaccination strategy. Scandinavian Journal of Infectious Diseases. 1996;**28**:217-224. DOI: 10.3109/00365549609027160

[59] Lotric-Furlan S, Strle F. Peripheral facial palsy in patients with tick-borne encephalitis. Clinical Microbiology and Infection. 2012;**18**:1027-1032. DOI: 1111/j.1469-0691.2011.03719.x

[60] Neumann B, Schulte-Mattler W, Brix S, Pöschl P, Jilg W, Bogdahn U, Steinbrecher A, Kleiter I. Autonomic and peripheral nervous system function in acute tick-borne encephalitis. Brain and Behavior. 2016;**6**:e00485. DOI: 10.1002/brb3.485

[61] Pöschl P, Kleiter I, Grubwinkler S, Bumes E, Bogdahn U, Dobler G, Steinbrecher A. Severe tick-borne encephalomyelitis with lack of cerebrospinal fluid pleocytosis (in German). Fortschritte Neurologie Psychiatrie. 2009;**77**:591-593. DOI: 10.1055/s-0028-1109768

[62] Stupica D, Strle F, Avšič-Županc T, Logar M, Pečavar B, Bajrović FF. Tick borne encephalitis without cerebrospinal fluid pleocytosis. BMC Infectious Diseases. 2014;**14**:614. DOI: 10.1186/s12879-014-0614-0

[63] Stiasny K, Holzmann H, Heinz FX. Characteristics of antibody responses in tick-borne encephalitis vaccination breakthroughs. Vaccine. 2009;**27**:7021-7026. DOI: 10.1016/j.vaccine.2009.09.069

[64] Andersson CR, Vene S, Insulander M, Lindquist L, Lundkvist A, Günther G. Vaccine failures after active immunisation against tick-borne encephalitis. Vaccine. 2010;**28**:2827-2831. DOI: 10.1016/j.vaccine.2010.02.001

[65] Zlamy M, Haberlandt E, Brunner J, Dozcy L, Rostasy K. Tick-borne encephalitis in a child with previous history of completed primary vaccination. Pediatrics International. 2016;**58**:56-58. DOI: 10.1111/ped.12752

[66] Kleiter I, Jilg W, Bogdahn U, Steinbrecher A. Delayed humoral immunity in a patient with severe tick-borne encephalitis after complete active vaccination. Infection. 2007;**35**:26-29. DOI: 10.1007/s15010-006-6614-2

[67] Lotric-Furlan, S, Avsic-Zupanc T, Strle F. Tick-borne encephalitis after active immunization. International Journal of Medical Microbiology. 2008;**298**(1):309-313. DOI: 10.1016/j.ijmm.2008.03.006

[68] Kunz C. TBE vaccination and the Austrian experience. Vaccine. 2003;**21**(Suppl 1): S50–S55. DOI: 10.1016/S0264-410X(02)00813-7

[69] Poponnikova TV. Specific clinical and epidemiological features of tick-borne encephalitis in Western Siberia. International Journal of Medical Microbiology. 2006;**296**(Suppl 40):59-62. DOI: 10.1016/j.ijmm.2006.01.023

[70] Khafizova IF, Iakupov EZ, Matveeva TV, Fazylov V, Ibatullin MM, Faizova AT, Khakimova AR, Mullaianova RF. The chronic form of tick-born encephalitis with a clinical manifestation of disseminated encephalomyelitis (case description) (in Russian). Zhurnal Nevrologii Psikhiatrii Imeni S S Korsakova. 2012;**112**:48-51

[71] Mukhin KY, Mameniskiene R, Mironov MB, Kvaskova NE, Bobylova MY, Petrukhin AS, Wolf P Epilepsia partialis continua in tick-borne Russian spring-summer encephalitis. Acta Neurologica Scandinavica. 2012;**125**:345-352. DOI: 10.1111/j.1600-0404.2011.01575.x

[72] Taba P, Lutsar I. Chronic infectious inflammatory diseases of the central nervous system. In: Deisenhammer F, Sellebjerg F, Teiunissen C, Tumani H, editors. Cerebrospinal Fluid in Clinical Neurology. Springer; Cham, Heidelberg, New York, Dordrecht, London 2015. pp. 211-245. DOI: 10.1007/978-3-319-01225-4_1

[73] Haglund M, Günther G. Tick-borne encephalitis-pathogenesis, clinical course and long-term follow-up. Vaccine. 2003;**21**(Suppl 1):S11–S18

[74] Misić Majerus L, Daković Rode O, Ruzić Sabljić E. Post-encephalitic syndrome in patients with tick-borne encephalitis (in Croatian). Acta Medica Croatica. 2009;**63**:269-278

[75] Kaiser R. Long term prognosis of patients with primary myelitic manifestation of tick-borne encephalitis: A trend analysis covering 10 years (in German). Nervenarzt. 2011;**82**:1020-1025. DOI: 10.1007/s00115-011-3254-2

[76] Veje M, Nolskog P, Petzold M, Bergström T, Lindén T, Peker Y, Studahl M. Tick-borne encephalitis sequelae at long-term follow-up: A self-reported case-control study. Acta Neurologica Scandinavica. 2016. DOI: 10.1111/ane.12561 [Epub ahead of print]

[77] Lotric-Furlan S, Petrovec M, Avsic-Zupanc T, Nicholson WL, Sumner JW, Childs JE, Strle F. Prospective assessment of the etiology of acute illness after a tick bite in Slovenia. Clinical Infectious Diseases. 2001;**33**:503-510. DOI: 10.1086/322586

[78] Lotric-Furlan S, Strle F. Trombocytopenia – A common finding in the initial phase of tick borne encephalitis. Infection. 1995;**23**:203-206. DOI: 10.1007/BF01781197

[79] Kaiser R, Holzmann H. Laboratory findings in tick-borne encephalitis – Correlation with clinical outcome. Infection. 2000;**28**:78-84. DOI: 10.1007/s150100050051

[80] Valdueza JM, Weber JR, Harms L, Bock A. Severe tick borne encephalomyelitis after tick bite and passive immunisation. Journal of Neurology, Neurosurgery, and Psychiatry. 1996;**60**:593-594

[81] Waldvogel K, Bossart W, Huisman T, Boltshauser E, Nadal D. Severe tick-borne encephalitis following passive immunization. European Journal of Pediatrics. 1996;**155**:775-779

[82] Vollmann H, Hagemann G, Mentzel HJ, Witte OW, Redecker C. Isolated reversible splenial lesion in tick-borne encephalitis: A case report and literature review. Clinical Neurology and Neurosurgery. 2011;**113**:430-433. DOI: 10.1016/j.clineuro.2011.01.010

[83] Severien C, Nachtrodt G, Teufel M. Frühsommermeningoenzephalitis bei einem Säugling. Mit Berücksichtigung der Erkrankungszahlen in Deutschland (Kasuistik). Tick-borne meningoencephalitis in an infant. Case report and overview (in German). Pädiatrische Praxis. 2011;**78**:95

[84] Ponfick M, Hacker S, Gdynia HJ, Linden R, Granz M, Nowak DA. Meningoencephaloradiculomyelitis after tick-borne encephalitis virus infection: A case series. European Journal of Neurology. 2012;**19**:776-782. DOI: 10.1111/j.1468-1331.2011.03651.x

[85] Bender A, Schulte-Altedorneburg G, Walther EU, Pfister HW. Severe tick borne encephalitis with simultaneous brain stem, bithalamic, and spinal cord involvement documented by MRI. Journal of Neurology, Neurosurgery, and Psychiatry. 2005;**76**:135-137. DOI: 10.1136/jnnp.2004.040469

[86] Alkadhi H, Kollias SS. MRI in tick-borne encephalitis. Neuroradiology. 2000;**42**:753-755

[87] Lorenzl S, Pfister HW, Padovan C, Yousry T. MRI abnormalities in tick-borne encephalitis. Lancet. 1996;**347**:698-699

[88] Pfister HW, Lorenzl S, Yousry T. Neuroradiographic manifestations of encephalitis. The New England journal of medicine. 1997;**337**:1393-1394. DOI: 10.1056/NEJM199711063371916

[89] Horger M, Beck R, Fenchel M, Ernemann U, Nägele T, Brodoefel H, Heckl S. Imaging findings in tick-borne encephalitis with differential diagnostic considerations. AJR American Journal of Roentgenology. 2012;**199**:420-427. DOI: 10.2214/AJR.11.7911

[90] Marjelund S, Tikkakoski T, Tuisku S, Räisänen S. Magnetic resonance imaging findings and outcome in severe tick-borne encephalitis. Report of Four Cases and Review of the Literature. Acta Radiologica. 2004;45:88-94

[91] Czupryna P, Tarasow E, Moniuszko-Malinowska A, Pancewicz S, Zajkowska O, Targoński A, Chorąży M, Rutkowski K, Dunaj J, Grygorczuk S, Kondrusik M, Zajkowska J. MRI and planimetric CT follow-up study of patients with severe tick-borne encephalitis. Infectious Diseases (London). 2016;**48**:74-81. DOI: 10.3109/23744235.2015.1083119

[92] Von Stülpnagel C, Winkler P, Koch J, Zeches-Kansy C, Schöttler-Glas A, Wolf G, Niller HH, Staudt M, Kluger G, Rostasy K. MRI-imaging and clinical findings of eleven children with tick-borne encephalitis and review of the literature. European Journal of Paediatric Neurology. 2016;**20**:45-52. DOI: 10.1016/j.ejpn.2015.10.008

[93] Rácz A, Schaller G, Lunkenheimer J, Engelhorn T, Dörfler A, Sperling W, Schwab S, Maihöfner C. Isolated meningomyeloradiculitis following infection with tick borne encephalitis virus. Clinical Neurology and Neurosurgery. 2012;114:1263-1265. DOI: 10.1016/j.clineuro.2012.02.047

[94] Stich O, Reinhard M, Rauer S. MRI scans of cervical cord provide evidence of anterior horn lesion in a patient with tick-borne encephalomyeloradiculitis. European Journal of Neurology. 2007;14:e5–e6. DOI: 10.1111/j.1468-1331.2007.01774.x

[95] Cruciatti B, Beltrame A, Ruscio M, Viale P, Gigli GL. Neurological manifestation of tick-borne encephalitis in North-Eastern Italy. Neurology Science. 2006;27:122-124. DOI: 10.1007/s10072-006-0612-0

[96] Pfefferkorn T, Feddersen B, Schulte-Altedorneburg G, Linn J, Pfister HW. Tick-borne encephalitis with polyradiculitis documented by MRI. Neurology. 2007;68:1232-1233. DOI: 10.1212/01.wnl.0000259065.58968.10

[97] Enzinger C, Melisch B, Reischl A, Simbrunner J, Fazekas F. Polyradiculitis as a predominant symptom of tick-borne encephalitis virus infection. Archives of Neurology. 2009;66:904-905. DOI: 10.1001/archneurol.2009.117

[98] Holzmann H. Diagnosis of tick-borne encephalitis. Vaccine. 2003;21(Suppl 1):S36–S40. DOI: 10.1016/S0264-410X(02)00819-8

[99] Ludolfs D, Reinholz M, Schmitz H. Highly specific detection of antibodies to tick-borne encephalitis (TBE) virus in human using domain III antigen and a sensitive immune complex (IC) ELISA. Journal of Clinical Virology. 2009;45:125-128. DOI: 10.1016/j.jcv.2009.03.016

[100] Günther G, Haglund M, Lindquist L, Sköldenberg B, Forsgren M. Intrathecal IgM, IgA and IgG antibody response in tick-borne encephalitis. Long-term follow-up related to clinical course and outcome. Clinical and Diagnostic Virology. 1997;8:17-29. DOI: 10.1016/S0928-0197(97)00273-0

[101] Hofmann H, Kunz C, Heinz FX, Dippe H. Detectability of IgM antibodies against TBE virus after natural infection and after vaccination. Infection. 1983;**11**:164-166. DOI: 10.1007/BF01641297

[102] Stiasny K, Aberle JH, Chmelik V, Karrer U, Holzmann H, Heinz FX. Quantitative determination of IgM antibodies reduces the pitfalls in the serodiagnosis of tick-borne encephalitis. Journal of Clinical Virology. 2012;54:115-120. DOI: 10.1016/j.jcv.2012.02.016

[103] Kaiser R. Tick-borne encephalitis – Still a serious disease? Wiener Medizinische Wochenschrift. 2012;162:229. DOI: 10.1007/s10354-012-0119-7

[104] Lesnicar G, Poljak M, Seme K, Lesnicar J. Pediatric tick-borne encephalitis in 371 cases from an endemic region in Slovenia, 1959 to 2000. The Pediatric Infectious Disease Journal. 2003;22:612-617. DOI: 10.1097/01.inf.0000073202.39700.a0

[105] Logar M, Arnez M, Kolbl J, Avsic-Zupanc T, Strle F. Comparison of the epidemiological and clinical features of tick-borne encephalitis in children and adults. Infection. 2000;28:74-77

[106] Kaiser R. Tick-borne encephalitis: Clinical findings and prognosis in adults. Wiener Medizinische Wochenschrift. 2012;162:239-243. DOI: 10.1007/s10354-012-0105-0

[107] Wahlberg P, Saikku P, Brummer-Korvenkontio M. Tick-borne viral encephalitis in Finland. The clinical features of Kumlinge disease during 1959-1987. Journal of Internal Medicine. 1989;225:173-177. DOI: 10.1111/j.1365-2796.1989.tb00059.x

[108] McNair AN, Brown JL. Tick-borne encephalitis complicated by monoplegia and sensorineural deafness. Journal of Infection. 1991;22:81-86. DOI: 10.1016/0163-4453(91)91094-E

[109] Anić K, Soldo I, Perić L, Karner I, Barac B. Tick-borne encephalitis in Eastern Croatia. Scandinavian Journal of Infectious Diseases. 1998;30:509-512. DOI: 10.1080/00365549850161548

[110] Jereb M, Muzlovic I, Avsic-Zupanc T, Karner P. Severe tick-borne encephalitis in Slovenia: Epidemiological, clinical and laboratory findings. Wiener Klinische Wochenschrift. 2002;114:623-626

[111] Tomazic J, Pikelj F, Schwartz B, Kunze M, Kraigher A, Matjašič M, Lesničar G, Gorišek J, Kunz C, Marth E, Slovenian TBE study group. The clinical features of tick-borne encephalitis in Slovenia. A study of 492 cases in 1994. Antibiotic Monitoring. 1996;12:115-120

[112] Logina I, Krumina A, Karelis G, Elsone L, Viksna L, Rozentale B, Donaghy M. Clinical features of double infection with tick-borne encephalitis and Lyme borreliosis transmitted by tick bite. Journal of Neurology, Neurosurgery, and Psychiatry. 2006;77:1350-1353. DOI: 10.1136/jnnp.2004.060731

[113] Cimperman J, Maraspin V, Lotric-Furlan S, Ruzić-Sabljić E, Avsic-Zupanc T, Picken RN, Strle F. Concomitant infection with tick-borne encephalitis virus and Borrelia burgdorferi sensu lato in patients with acute meningitis or meningoencephalitis. Infection. 1998;26:160-164

[114] Kindberg E, Mickiene A, Ax C, Åkerlind B, Vene S, Lindquist L, Lundkvist Å, Svensson L. A deletion in the chemokine receptor 5 (CCR5) gene is associated with tick-borne encephalitis. Clinical Infectious Diseases. 2008;197:266-269. DOI: 10.1086/524709

[115] Kindberg E, Vene S, Mickiene A, Lundkvist Å, Lindquist L, Svensson L. A functional Toll-like receptor 3 gene (TLR3) may be a risk factor for tick-borne encephalitis virus (TBEV) infection. Journal of Infectious Dieseases. 2011;203:523-528. DOI: 10.1093/infdis/jiq082

[116] Mickiene A, Pakalniene J, Nordgren J, Carlsson B, Hagbom M, Svensson L, Lindquist L. Polymorphisms in chemokine receptor 5 and Toll-like receptor 3 genes are risk factors for clinical tick-borne encephalitis in the Lithuanian population. PLoS One. 2014;9:e106798. DOI: 10.1371/journal.pone.0106798

[117] Barkhash AV, Perelygin AA, Babenko VN, Brinton MA, Voevoda MI. Single nucleotide polymorphism in the promoter region of the CD209 gene is associated with human predisposition to severe forms of tick-borne encephalitis. Antiviral Research. 2012;93:64-68. DOI: 10.1016/j.antiviral.2011.10.017

[118] Barkhash AV, Perelygin AA, Babenko VN, Myasnikova NG, Pilipenko PI, Romaschenko AG, Voevoda MI, Brinton MA. Variability in the 2'-5'-oligoadenylate synthetase gene cluster is associated with human predisposition to tick-borne encephalitis virus-induced disease. Journal of Infectious Diseases. 2010;202:1813-1818. DOI: 10.1086/657418

[119] Lotric-Furlan S, Petrovec M, Avsic-Zupanc T, Logar M, Strle F. Epidemiological, clinical and laboratory distinction between human granulocytic ehrlichiosis and the initial phase of tick-borne encephalitis. Wiener Klinische Wochenschrift. 2002;114:636-640

[120] Kristoferitsch W, Stanek G, Kunz C. Doppelinfektion mit Fruhsommermeningo-enzephalitis (FSME) virus und Borrelia burgdorferi (in German). Deutsche Medizinische Wochenschrift. 1987;111:861-864. DOI: 10.1055/s-2008-1068546

[121] Oksi J, Viljanen MK, Kalimo H, Peltonen R, Marttia R, Salomaa P, Nikoskelainen J, Budka H, Halonen P. Fatal encephalitis caused by concomitant infection with tick-borne encephalitis virus and Borrelia burgdorferi. Clinical Infectious Diseases. 1993;16:392-396. DOI: 10.1093/clind/16.3.392

[122] Lotric-Furlan S, Petrovec M, Avsic-Zupanc T, Strle F. Concomitant tick-borne encephalitis and human granulocytic ehrlichiosis. Emerging Infectious Diseases. 2005;11:485-488. DOI: 10.3201/eid1103.040776

[123] Kneen R, Solomon T, Appleton R. The role of lumbar puncture in suspected CNS infection – A disappearing skill? Archives of Disease in Childhood. 2002;87:181-183

[124] Kramer AH. Viral encephalitis in the ICU. Critical Care Clinics. 2013;29:621-649. DOI: 10.1016/j.ccc.2013.03.011

[125] Lani R, Moghaddam E, Haghani A, Chang LY, AbuBakar S, Zandi K. Tick-borne viruses: A review from the perspective of therapeutic approaches. Ticks and Tick-Borne Diseases. 2014;**5**:457-465. DOI: 10.1016/j.ttbdis.2014.04.001

[126] Czupryna P, Moniuszko A, Pancewicz SA, Grygorczuk S, Kondrusik M, Zajkowska J. Tick-borne encephalitis in Poland in years 1993-2008 – Epidemiology and clinical presentation. A retrospective study of 687 patients. European Journal of Neurology. 2011;18:673-679. DOI: 10.1111/j.1468-1331.2010.03278.x

[127] Vazquez M, Muehlenbein C, Cartter M, Hayes EB, Ertel S, Shapiro ED. Effectiveness of personal protective measures to prevent Lyme disease. Emerging Infectious Diseases. 2008;14:210-216. DOI: 10.3201/eid1402.070725

[128] Corapi KM, White MI, Phillips CB, Daltroy LH, Shadick NA, Liang MH. Strategies for primary and secondary prevention of Lyme disease. Nature Clinical Practice Rheumatology. 2007;3:20-25. DOI: 10.1038/ncprheum0374

[129] Kluger G, Schöttler A, Waldvogel K, Nadal D, Hinrichs W, Wündisch GF, Laub MC. Tick-borne encephalitis despite specific immunoglobulin prophylaxis. Lancet. 1995;346:1502. DOI: 10.1016/S0140-6736(95)92527-9

[130] Bröker M, Kollaritsch H. After a tick bite in a tick-borne encephalitis virus endemic area: Current positions about post-exposure treatment. Vaccine. 2008;26:863-868. DOI: 10.1016/j.vaccine.2007.11.046

[131] Barrett PN, Porthsmouth D, Ehrlich HJ. Tick-borne encephalitis virus vaccines. In: Plotkin SA, Orenstein W, Offit PA, editors. Vaccines. 6th ed. Elsevier; Philadelphia, PA 2013. pp. 773-788

[132] Pen'evskaia NA, Rudakov NV. Efficiency of use of immunoglobulin preparations for the postexposure prevention of tick-borne encephalitis in Russia (a review of semi-centennial experience) (in Russian). Meditsinskaia Parazitologiia (Mosk). 2010;1:53-59

[133] WHO. Vaccines against tick-borne encephalitis: WHO position paper. Weekly Epidemiology Record. 2011;86:241-256

[134] Haditsch M, Kunze U. Tick-borne encephalitis: A disease neglected by travel medicine. Travel Medicine and Infectious Disease. 2013;11:295-300. DOI: 10.1016/j.tmaid.2013.07.003

[135] Zavadska D, Anca I, André F, Bakir M, Chlibek R, Cižman M, Ivaskeviciene I, Mangarov A, Mészner Z, Pokorn M, Prymula R, Richter D, Salman N, Simurka P, Tamm E, Tešović G, Urbancikova I, Usonis V. Recommendations for tick-borne encephalitis vaccination from the Central European Vaccination Awareness Group (CEVAG). Human Vaccines & Immunotherapeutics. 2013;9:362-374. DOI: 10.4161/hv.22766

[136] Wiedermann U. Tick borne encephalitis TBE – Vaccination in non-endemic countries. Travel Medicine and Infectious Disease. 2010;8:251-256. DOI: 10.1016/j.tmaid.2010.05.007

[137] Schöndorf I, Schönfeld C, Nicolay U, Zent O, Banzhoff A. Response to tick-borne encephalitis (TBE) booster vaccination after prolonged time intervals to primary immunization with the rapid schedule. International Journal of Medical Microbiology. 2006;**296**(Suppl 40):S208–S212. DOI: 10.1016/j.ijmm.2006.01.009

[138] Heinz FX, Stiasny K, Holzmann H, Grgic-Vitek M, Kriz B, Essl A, Kundi M. Vaccination and tick-borne encephalitis, Central Europe. Emerging Infectious Diseases. 2013;19:69-76. DOI: 10.3201/eid1901.120458

Chapter 4

Herpes Meningoencephalitis: Causes, Diagnosis, and Treatment

Sandip Kumar Dash

Additional information is available at the end of the chapter

http://dx.doi.org/10.5772/intechopen.68553

Abstract

Meningoencephalitis also known as encephalomeningitis is an inflammation of the brain and its surrounding protective membranes. It resembles both meningitis and encephalitis. Meningoencephalitis can be caused by bacteria, viruses, fungi, and protozoan or as secondary sequel of other inflammations like AIDS. The viral or aseptic meningoencephalitis is mainly caused by enteroviruses, varicella-zoster viruses, herpes simplex viruses, or measles viruses. Among the various causes of viral meningoencephalitis, herpes meningoencephalitis (HME), caused by herpes simplex virus type 1 and 2, is dreadful. It is a communicable infection spread through droplets, air, water, food, sexual intercourse, or effected mother to child. The symptoms of the disease resemble to common viral infections except few like nuchal rigidity, blurred vision, and purple body rashes. Diagnosis is carried out from body fluids like urine, saliva, blood, or cerebrospinal fluid using laboratory methods, imaging techniques, PCR or enzyme-linked immunosorbent assays. The causes, diagnosis, prevention, and treatments of HME are discussed detail in this chapter.

Keywords: encephalitis, encephalomeningitis, herpes meningoencephalitis, meninges, meningitis, meningoencephalitis

1. Introduction

Mammalian brain and spinal cords are covered by three membranous tissue layers pia mater, arachnoid mater, and dura mater (from inner to outer) forming meninges. Infection in these layers is known as meningitis. An inflammation or infection in the brain tissue is known as encephalitis [1]. The infection in the brain and meninges together is known as meningoencephalitis or encephalomeningitis. This can be caused by either of the bacteria, fungi, viruses, or protozoans. Viral or aseptic meningoencephalitis, caused by herpes simplex virus type 1 (HSV 1) and 2 (HSV 2), is known as herpes meningoencephalitis (HME) [2]. The direct infection in the brain or meninges is called primary HME, whereas if it spreads from other parts to the brain, then it is called secondary HME. Both the male and female are affected at an equal ratio with a higher mortality and morbidity rate (~50%) for infants. Like a communicable infection, spread through air, water, or close contact [3], the viruses after entering the patient through mouth, nose, or genital tract reach to the brain-crossing blood-brain barrier and cause infection.

The symptoms of this infection are a combinatorial effect of both the meningitis and encephalitis insisting the physicians to suspect meningoencephalitis [4]. Symptoms resemble to the common viral infections but may vary among the children and adults. Some of the typical symptoms of HME are nuchal rigidity, blurred vision, and purple body rashes. The infection can spread among people through droplets, foods, air, or close contact. There is always a need for early diagnosis of the infection followed by treatment. The disease can be suspected initially on the basis of the specific symptoms of the patients. This can be further confirmed by several laboratory-based, imaging, or advanced techniques [5]. Although the prevention of HME is not possible through vaccination, but proper precaution measures can reduce the risk of spreading and relapsing of the disease. Abstain or safety measures during sexual intercourse and proper management during pregnancy lessen the risk of contamination.

Mild infected persons may recover in few weeks but a severely infected person requires longer time and intense care. Early treatment of the patients with antiviral drugs may hugely reduce the risk of the contamination and death. Anticonvulsants or diuretics can minimize the inflammation, cranial pressure, or pain. In this chapter, we have discussed in detail about the symptoms, causes, diagnosis, prevention, and treatment of HME.

2. Symptoms

The symptoms of HME resemble to common flu and may vary among children, adults, and neonates. HME type 1 is more prominent at age below 20 years or over 40 years. The earlier symptoms shown in children and adults are fever, disorientation, or speech problem. At a later stage, headache, vomiting, fever, drowsiness, seizures, and unconsciousness also appear. Specific symptoms of this infection are nuchal rigidity, blurred vision, hallucinations, purple rashes or behavioral changes [4]. Infants are mainly infected by type 2, and the symptoms include high fever, bulging of forehead, poor feeding or constant sleepiness.

3. Causes

HME is mainly caused by HSV type 1, type 2 or as secondary squeal of other diseases like Crohn's disease [2, 6]. HME accounts for about 10% of the total meningoencephalitis cases with a effecting rate of about $2/10^6$. Most of the HME cases are seen in case of infants or children. The infection is contaminated through coughing, sneezing or close contact. Type 1 viruses can spread through food, water, and air, whereas type 2 transmits mainly through sexual contact [3]. Sometimes, after complete treatment, also the viruses remain silently in the body and relapse at a later stage. AIDS, alcoholism, diabetes, immunosuppressant drugs, splenectomy, and other immunosuppressive factors increase the susceptibility of a person toward getting infected. The infection may cause partial or complete impairment of the brain or sensory organs, kidney failure or death [7]. Therefore, there is a compulsory need for an early diagnosis of the disease followed by treatment.

4. Diagnosis

On the basis of different symptoms seen in the suspected patients, physicians suggest different preliminary or confirmatory diagnostic tests [5]. Diagnosis of the HME involves several stages, initially differentiation from other closely related infections and then distinguishes between bacterial, fungal, and viral meningoencephalitis. The final step involves confirmation of HME from other forms of aseptic meningoencephalitis. Diagnosis can be carried out from blood, saliva, urine or cerebrospinal fluid (CSF) of the patients with the CSF being preference. Diagnosis of HME is done as below:

4.1. Laboratory methods

4.1.1. Body fluid test

Different types of body fluids like urine, blood, or saliva of the suspected patients can be tested for antigens, antibodies, level of WBCs, proteins, procalcitonin, or glucose. These components are mainly detected through biochemical analysis or immunological assays. Increase in the WBC count in the CSF or the presence of IgM antibodies in the serum confirm HME. The level of these components confirms pathogenic condition of a person and differentiates between bacterial, fungal, and aseptic meningoencephalitis. The presence of WBCs or microorganisms turns the CSF from transparent to cloudy in color. Increase in the lymphocyte count is a characteristic of viral infection. Increase in the amount of proteins or decrease in the glucose in CSF also confirm viral infection. But biochemical analysis may be inconclusive or misleading. Therefore, further tests like PCR or blotting must be carried out for further confirmation of the specific infection. Sometimes, the samples from the patients are cultured and sensitivity tests carried out for confirmation of the pathogen [8–10]. But this consumes 2–3 days for confirmation. Microscopic analysis of the patient samples is also another alternative diagnostic method. But this is a preliminary mode of diagnosis and nonspecific.

4.1.2. Spinal tap

Diagnosis using CSF through spinal tap or lumbar puncture is one of the most preferable methods to distinguish meningoencephalitis from blood toxicity or sepsis. This technique involves extraction of about 0.5–1.0 ml of CSF from the subarachnoid space between lumbar (L) vertebrae L3/L4 or L4/L5 [8]. The change in the composition of CSF, presence of pathogens or their by-products, presence of lactic acid, lactate dehydrogenase, or C-reactive proteins or increase in the white blood cells (WBCs) count of CSF can be detected by various methods [9, 10]. CSF-based detection is one of the traditional methods used for the diagnosis of several disorders associated with the central nervous system. Although the method is less time consuming, it is low sensitivity and nonspecific.

4.2. Non-laboratory tests

4.2.1. Electroencephalography

This is a noninvasive electrophysiological technique which analyze the electrical signals or ionic current within the neurons of the brain. Any abnormalities or functional changes in the brain cause change in neural oscillation or brain waves over a period of time which can be detected [11]. The pattern of the waves in an electroencephalogram signifies the specific type of seizure or viral infection [12]. Despite its low resolution, it is still used as one of the pioneer diagnostic tool. This method consumes several hours for complete detection of the pathogen.

4.2.2. Neurological examinations

HME may cause partial or complete impairment of the brain and the sensory system in the patient. Therefore, physician carries out neurological examinations to confirm the infection. Neurological examination is carried out through series of tests to detect neurological disorders, mental status, strengths of sensation, and behavioral changes. Simple instruments like forks, reflex hammer, or small pins are used by the physicians to detect the strength of the neurological response. But this test is nonspecific and misleading because it cannot discriminate between HME and meningocephalitis due to other causes.

4.3. Radiological methods

4.3.1. CT scan

Use of CT scan has gained preference over other methods during last few decades for diagnosis [13, 14]. CT scan or X-ray CT involves two dimensional X-ray images of the brain from several possible angles and computer-based analysis for any deformities. Sometimes, dyes are also used to differentially highlight the different parts of brain [15]. This technique clearly visualizes any type of blood hemorrhage, clot, swellings, infections, or inflammations in the brain or the meninges. The dark areas signify for edema, whereas bright areas signify calcification or hemorrhage of the brain tissue. Although the high resolution of CT scan proved it to be better diagnostics method over others conventional methods but is associated with several side effects like damaging tissue and cancer. Therefore, is less preferred in the case of infants or children.

4.3.2. MRI-based detection

Since 1970, after discovery, MRI is used as one of most versatile and prominent diagnostic tool in biomedical research. MRI or NMRI uses magnetic fields, radio waves, and field gradients to image the anatomy or physiological structure of brain [16]. A clear image obtained there of reveals any infection or inflammation in the brain or meninges. Since, this technique does not use any ionizing radiations and has a higher sensitivity, therefore, preferred over CT scan. This method is sometimes time-consuming, expensive, and cumbersome [17].

4.3.3. *Brain biopsy*

This technique involves digging a hole at a point in the skull identified through CT scan or MRI, collection of small tissue using sterilized needle, and then observation under microscope [18]. The status or condition of the brain and its surrounding tissue can be analyzed through this method. HME is detected depending upon the swelling or damage of the tissue. This method although is highly sensitive but painful and associated with several complications. Therefore, this method was slowly replaced by other methods.

4.3.4. *Ultrasound*

Ultrasound or sonography is a nondestructive method uses sound wave of >20 kHz to study the structure and secretions from brain. These wave with very short wavelength and low power density resolute every change in the brain without heating or cavitations effect [19]. Infection, swelling, lesions, or inflammation of the brain or the associated tissue can be clearly imaged. Despite these, over exposure to this wave may cause side effects like hearing loss and organ dysfunction.

4.4. Future directions

A quick and specific diagnosis of any disease is necessary to initiate an early treatment against it. Present diagnostic methods for HME are inconclusive, time-consuming, misleading, non-specific, or complicated. Therefore, there is a need for a quick, simple, sensitive, and specific method for diagnosis of HME. Nowadays, several advanced methods have been developed for the diagnosis of different types of diseases. The principles of these methods can be used to develop a quick, simple, and reliable diagnostic method in future. Detection of any pathogen based on the analysis of partial or complete genome is one of the most preferred techniques nowadays. The genome of HSV is approximately of 152 kb which can be very easily analyzed as below:

4.4.1. *PCR*

Since the discovery of PCR, it is used as quick, specific, and sensitive method for diagnosis of several diseases. Several researchers proposed PCR-based detection of HSV from patient samples through designing specific primers and found higher sensitive than other conventional methods [5, 20–22]. The PCR amplicons can be analyzed which is an agarose gel electrophoresis with or without Southern blotting [23], although Southern blotting increases the sensitivity of a PCR but increase the time taken. Therefore, some researchers replaced it with enzyme-linked inmmunosorbent assay. Recently, we have reported very less time-consuming direct PCR for detection of *Neisseria meningitidis* from the CSF samples (**Figure 1**) [24, 25]. The same procedure may be followed to detect HSV in future.

4.4.2. Biosensors

Biosensors are replacing the traditional diagnostic methods because of their sensitivity, specificity, simplicity, and economical value [26–29]. A biosensor contains a biotransducer or bioreceptor which interact with the analyte, and the signal released is detected by a detector. At a low analyte concentration, electrochemical sensor is more favorable than the others (**Figure 2**) [28, 29]. For construction of an electrochemical sensor, ionic bonding between the gold and thiol-group can be used for immobilization. Which can be further hybridized with the complementary analyte and detected electrochemically (**Figure 3**) [28, 29]. Metallic nanoparticles and carbon nanotubes can also be used to increase the surface of immobilization and sensitivity of the sensor for quick, sensitive, and specific diagnosis of large number of HME suspected samples at a time [30, 31].

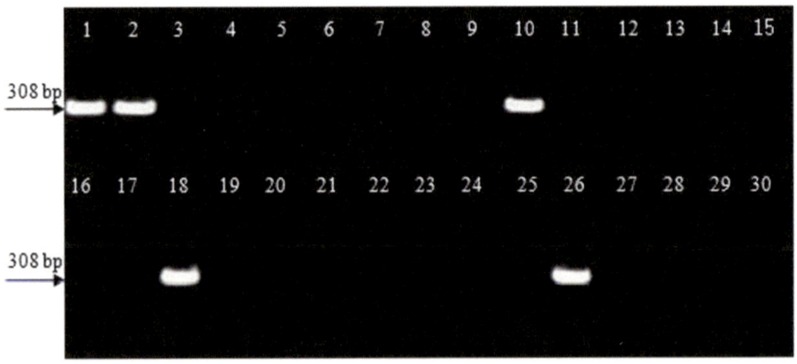

Figure 1. PCR-based diagnosis of bacterial meningitis Lane 1 and 2: control, lane 10, 16, and 26: infected patients, and lane 3-9, 11-15, 17-25, and 12-20: negative [25].

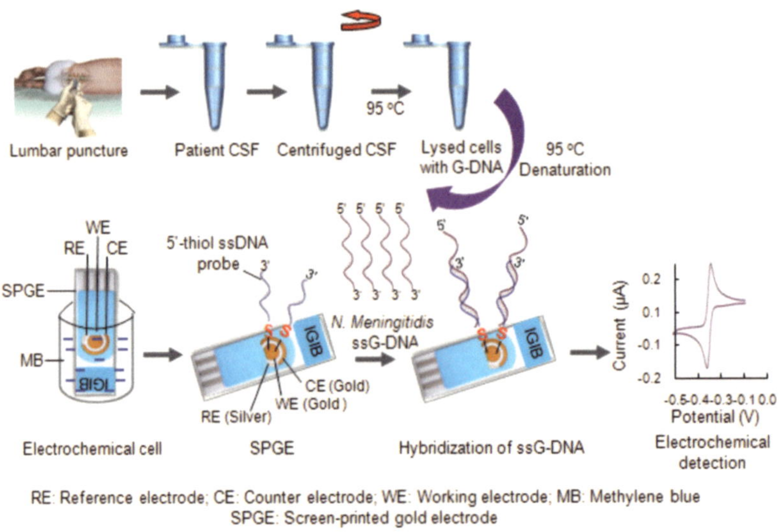

Figure 2. Schematic representation of immobilization of thiol-labeled probe onto gold electrode and detection of *N. meningitidis* from patient CSF [29].

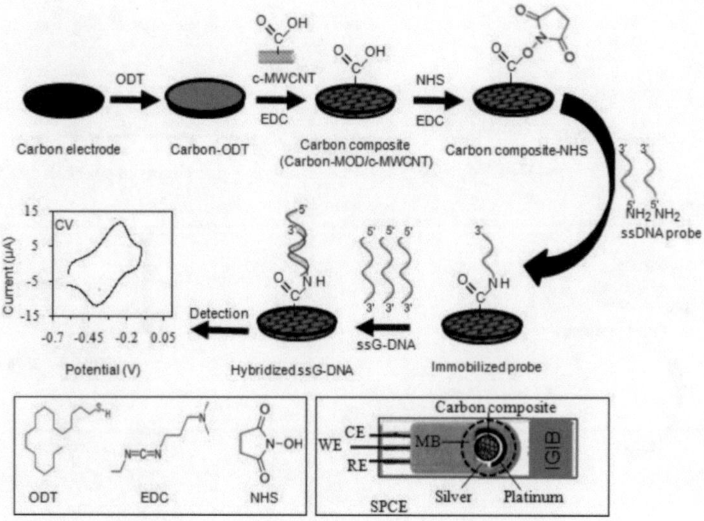

Figure 3. Schematic representation of immobilization of probe on nanocomposite and diagnosis of bacterial meningitis from patient CSF [30].

4.4.3. *Microarray*

Microarray involves immobilization of an array of single or multiple types of ssDNA probes onto a surface and then hybridization with complementary ssDNA followed by detection through LASER scanning. Microarray is an advance and promising technique for diagnosis of any disease [32]. Tong et al. first time used 16S microarray for detection of neonatal bacterial meningitis using patient's blood [33]. Nowadays, DNA microarray is used for detection of large number of suspected samples of different diseases at a time. DNA microarray can either be constructed by direct synthesis of oligonucleotide on the solid surface (affymetrix microarray) or by immobilization of earlier synthesized oligonucleotides onto a substrate [34]. The second one remains as choice of preference for the researchers because of its flexibility regarding the surface and ligand used for construction of microarray [35]. Glasses are preferred over other platforms due to their low-cost, intrinsic fluorescence, and superior optical properties. 3′-modified probe is preferred over the 5′-modified probe because the later requires phosphoramidite reagents of the modifier in strictly anhydrous condition [36]. Surface of the substrates can be coated with polylysine or aminopropyle to increase the immobilization. The noncovalent attachments used for immobilization of the ssDNA probe onto an electrode are epoxide-amine, epoxide-thiol, epoxide-aminooxyalkyl, aldehyde-amine, and semicarbazide-aldehyde. Carboxyl-amine, thiol-disulfide, biotin-streptavidin, gold-thiol, zirconylated-surface-phosphate, and epoxide-amine are some of the covalent linkage used often for the probe immobilization (**Figure 4**) [34]. The immobilization of the probe is optimized for time, pH, temperature, and concentration in order to obtain maximum immobilization efficiency. The array of immobilized oligomers can be hybridized with the genomic DNA of pathogen in patient sample. Several researches have been reported by our lab to detect the presence of *N. meningitidis* from the CSF samples using microarray [35, 36]. The same principle can be used to develop a microchip in future for diagnosis of large number of HME suspected samples at a time.

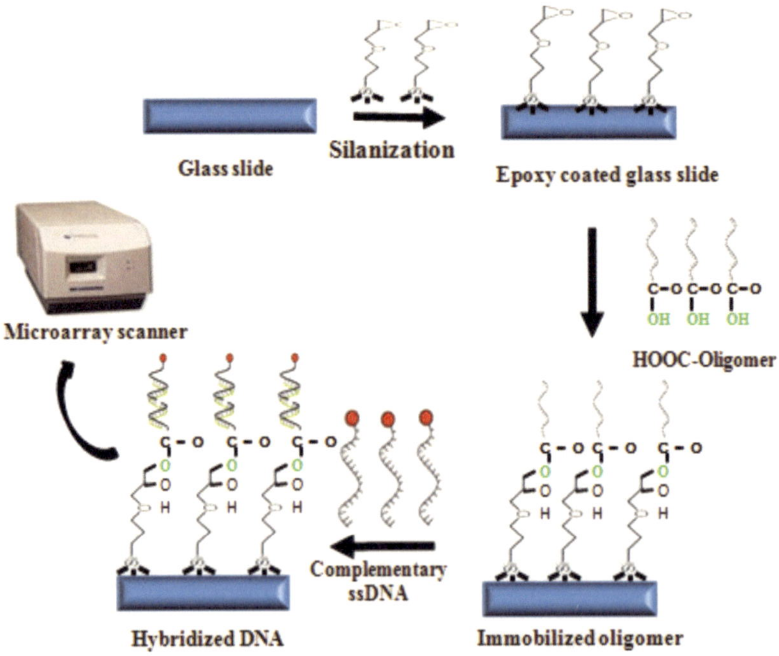

Figure 4. Schematic presentation of microarray-based detection of bacterial meningitis [35].

5. Prevention

It has always been said that prevention is better than cure. There is no effective vaccine available against HME, but prevention lies primarily in the management of genital infections in pregnant women [37]. Avoiding of sharing of food, beverages, and other objects in between the infected and healthy persons prevent the contamination of HME. Proper cleaning, sterilization, sanitation, and isolation also help to prevent spread of the infection [38]. Regular monitoring and health checkups are necessary for the people living in mass, working together, or pilgrims to avoid the risk of contaminations. Abstain from sex or protected sexual relation through latex condoms can reduce the risk of sexual transmission.

6. Treatment

Patients suffering with mild infection recover within few weeks of treatment, whereas severe cases may require longer period. About 50–70% of the HME patients suffer from secondary sequel-like brain damage, neurological disorders or comma. Therefore, an early treatment of the HME is necessary [39]. A dramatic improvement in the HME patient health can be achieved by treating at an earlier stage with antiviral drugs like acyclovir, vidarabine, or famciclovir. At a later stage, the treatment becomes ineffective. Anticonvulsants such as dilantin or phenytoin prevent HME seizures [40]. Corticosteroids or diuretics such as prednisone, furosemide, or mannitol can relieve the skull pressure, reduce swelling due to inflammation, and prevent hearing loss. In the case of severe inflammations, pain suppressors or sedatives may be prescribed. Complete rehabilitation, rest, regular monitoring, balanced nutrition, and occupational therapy are necessary for preventing relapse of the infection.

7. Conclusions

HME is one of the most dreadful forms of aseptic meningoencephalitis caused by HSV 1 and 2. It has a high mortality and morbidity rate especially in infants. The fail to accurate diagnosis and complete treatment has raised the risk of disease. Therefore, a rapid and accurate diagnosis is essential for early treatment of the infection and effective public health management. The inefficacy for eradication of any disease is equally shared by ignorance of the people and fail of early treatment. Therefore, the dreadful impact of this disease should be made aware to the common people. Recent advances in the field of diagnosis such as PCR, microarray, and nanosensors may help for early diagnosis. Still, there is a high demand on the research regarding early treatment of the infection to save the life of people.

Acknowledgements

I would like to thank Mrs. Sanjukta Satapthy, Principal, Chikiti College, Ganjam for her suggestions and advises.

Author details

Sandip Kumar Dash

Address all correspondence to: dashsandipkumar@gmail.com

Chikiti College, Chikiti, Odisha, India

References

[1] Kelly TA, Olorcain P, Moran J, Garvey P, McKeown P, Connell J, et al. Underreporting of viral encephalitis and viral meningitis, Ireland, 2005-2008. Emerging Infectious Diseases. 2013;**19**:1428-1436

[2] Tyler KL. Herpes simplex virus infections of the central nervous system: Encephalitis and meningitis, including Mollaret's. Herpes. 2004;**2**:57A-64A

[3] Tunkel AR, Glaser CA, Bloch KC, Sejvar JJ, Marra CM, Roos KL, et al. The management of encephalitis: Clinical practice guidelines by the Infectious Diseases Society of America. Clinical Infectious Diseases. 2008;**47**:303-327

[4] Ghaziuddin M, Al-Khouri I, Ghaziuddin N. Autistic symptoms following herpes encephalitis. European Child Adolescent Psychiatry. 2002;**11**:142-146

[5] Lakeman FD, Whitley RJ. Diagnosis of herpes simplex encephalitis: Application of polymerase chain reaction to cerebrospinal fluid from brain-biopsied patients and correlation with disease. The Journal of Infectious Diseases. 1995;**171**:857-863

[6] Robineau O, Enrico J, Lemaire L, Poissy J, Legout L, Senneville E, et al. Herpes simplex virus meningoencephalitis in a patient with Crohn's disease on azathioprine therapy. The American Journal of Gasteroeneterology. 2010;**105**:240-241

[7] Bruyn HB, Sexton HM, Brainerd HD. Mumps meningoencephalitis: A clinical review of 119 cases with one death. California Medicine. 1957;**86**:153-160

[8] Lopez T, Sanchez FJ, Garzon JC, Muriel C. Spinal anesthesia in pediatric patients. Minerva Anestesiologica. 2012;**78**:78-87

[9] Visintin C, Mugglestone MA, Fields EJ, Jacklin P, Murphy MS, Pollard AJ. Management of bacterial meningitis and meningococcal septicaemia in children and young people: Summary of NICE guidance. British Medical Journal. 2010;**340**:c3209

[10] Casasoprana A, Hachon Le Camus C, Claudet I, Grouteau E, Chaix Y, Cances C, et al. Value of lumbar puncture after a first febrile seizure in children aged less than 18 months. Archives de Pédiatrie. 2013;**20**:594-600

[11] Niedermeyer E, da Silva FL, editors. Electroencephalography: Basic Principles, Clinical Applications, and Related Fields. 6th ed. Lippincot Williams Wilkins; 2004. p. 1243

[12] Tinmaswala MA, Valinjker SK, Hegde S, Taware P. Electroencephalographic abnormalities in first onset afebrile and complex febrile seizures and its association with type of seizures. Journal of Medical Science and Clinical Research. 2015;**3**:7073-7082

[13] Semelka RC, Armao DM, Elias J, Huda W. Imaging strategies to reduce the risk of radiation in CT studies, including selective substitution with MRI. Journal of Magnetic Resonance Imaging. 2007;**25**:900-909

[14] Tubiana M. Comment on computed tomography and radiation exposure. The New England Journal of Medicine. 2008;**358**:852-853

[15] Hasbun R, Abrahams J, Jekel J, Quagliarello VJ. Computed tomography of the head before lumbar puncture in adults with suspected meningitis. The New England Journal of Medicine. 2001;**345**:1727-1733

[16] Heeger DJ, Ress D. What does fMRI tell us about neuronal activity?. Nature Reviews Neuroscience. 2002;**3**:142-151

[17] Hollingworth W, Todd CJ, Bell MI, Arafat Q, Girling S, Karia KR, Dixon AK. The diagnostic and therapeutic impact of MRI: An observational multi-centre study. Clinical Radiology. 2000;**55**:825-831

[18] Biopsy. American Brain Tumor Association. [Internet]. 2013. Available from: http://www.abta.org/understanding-brain-tumors/diagnosis/biopsy.html

[19] Pollet B, editor. Power Ultrasound in Electrochemistry: From Versatile Laboratory Tool to Engineering Solution. Wiley; 2012. p. 364

[20] Cinque P, Cleator GM, Weber T, Monteyne P, Sindic CJ, van Loon AM. The role of laboratory investigation in the diagnosis and management of patients with suspected herpes simplex encephalitis: A consensus report. Journal of Neurology, Neurosurgery, and Psychiatry. 1996;**61**:339-345

[21] Kimura H, Shibata M, Kuzushima K, Nishikawa K, Nishiyama Y, Morishima T. Detection and direct typing of herpes simplex virus by polymerase chain reaction. Medical Microbiology and Immunology. 1990;**179**:177-184

[22] Aslanzadeh J, Osmon DR, Wilhelm MP, Espy MJ, Smith TF. A prospective study of the polymerase chain reaction for detection of herpes simplex virus in cerebrospinal fluid submitted to the clinical virology laboratory. Molecular and Cellular Probes. 1992;**6**:367-373

[23] Tang Y-W, Mitchell PS, Espy MJ, Smith TF, Persing DH. Molecular diagnosis of herpes simplex virus infections in the central nervous system. Journal of Clinical Microbiology. 1999;**37**:2127-2136

[24] Dash SK, Sharma M, Khare S, Kumar A. *rmpM* gene as a genetic marker for human bacterial meningitis. Cellular and Molecular Biology. 2012;**58**:26-30

[25] Dash SK, Sharma M, Khare S, Kumar A. Quick diagnosis of human brain meningitis using *Omp85* gene amplicon as a genetic marker. Indian Journal of Microbiology. 2013;**53**:238-240

[26] Patel MK, Solanki PR, Kumar A, Khare S, Gupta S, Malhotra BD. Electrochemical DNA sensor for *Neisseria meningitidis* detection. Biosensors and Bioelectronics. 2010;**25**: 2586-2591

[27] Dash SK, Sharma M, Kumar A. Diagnostic techniques and treatment of meningitis. In: Houllis G, Karachalios M, editors. Meningitis: Causes, Diagnosis and Treatment. Nova Science Publishers Inc.; 2012. pp. 203-223

[28] Dash SK, Sharma M, Khare S, Kumar A. *Omp85* DNA sensor for detection of human brain bacterial meningitis. Biotechnology Letters. 2013;**35**:929-935

[29] Dash SK, Sharma M, Khare S, Kumar A. *rmpM* DNA sensor for detection of human brain bacterial meningitis in cerebrospinal fluid. Applied Biochemistry and Biotechnology. 2013;**171**:198-208

[30] Dash SK, Sharma M, Khare S, Kumar A. Carbon-mercaptooctadecane/carboxylated multi-walled carbon nanotubes composite based genosensor for detection of bacterial meningitis. Indian Journal of Microbiology. 2014;**54**:170-177

[31] Dash SK, Sharma M, Kumar A, Khare S, Kumar A. Carbon composite-based DNA sensor for detection of bacterial meningitis caused by *N. meningitidis*. Journal of Solid State Electrochemistry. 2014;**18**:2647-2659

[32] Sethi D, Kumar A, Gupta, KC, and Kumar P. A facile method for the construction of oligonucleotides microarrays. Bioconjugate Chemistry. 2008;**19**;2136-2143

[33] Tong M, Shang S, Wu Y, Zhao Z. Value of 16S RNA microarray detection in early diagnosis of neonatal septicemia. World Journal of Pediatrics. 2005;**2**:121-126

[34] Mahajan S, Sethi D, Seth S, Kumar A, Kumar P, Gupta KC. Construction of oligonucleotides microarrays (biochips) via thioether linkage for the detection of bacterial meningitis. Bioconjugate Chemistry. 2009;**20**:1703-1710

[35] Sethi D, Kumar A, Gandhi RP, Kumar P, Gupta KC. New protocol for oligonucleotide microarray fabrication using SU-8-coated glass microslides. Bioconjugate Chemistry. 2010;**211**:703-708

[36] Patnaik S, Dash SK, Sethi D, Kumar A, Gupta KC, Kumar P. Engineered polymer-supported synthesis of 3'-carboxyalkyl-modified oligonucleotides and their applications in the construction of biochips for diagnosis of the diseases. Bioconjugate Chemistry. 2012;**23**:664-670

[37] Nigrovic LE, Fine AM, Monuteaux MC, Shah SS, Neuman MI. Trends in the management of viral meningitis at United States children's hospitals. Pediatrics. 2013;**131**:670-676

[38] Landry ML, Greenwold J, Vikram HR. Herpes simplex type-2 meningitis: Presentation and lack of standardized therapy. American Journal of Medicine. 2009;**122**:688-691

[39] Alexandra L. Diagnosis and treatment of viral meningitis. AMA Journal of Ethics. 2007;**9**:497-498

[40] Desmond RA, Accortt NA, Talley L, Villano SA, Soong SJ, Whitley RJ. Enteroviral meningitis: Natural history and outcome of pleconaril therapy. Antimicrobial Agents and Chemotherapy. 2006;**50**:2409-2414

Chapter 5

Scrub Typhus Meningoencephalitis

Masaraf Hussain

Additional information is available at the end of the chapter

http://dx.doi.org/10.5772/intechopen.68369

Abstract

Scrub typhus is a zoonotic disease, which is characterized by an acute febrile illness, lymphadenopathy, eschar, multisystem involvement, and a rapid response to doxycycline. It is found widely in Asia and Pacific islands. Various neurological manifestations, like meningoencephalitis, cranial nerve involvement, are known to occur. Diagnosis is based on a high clinical suspicion, presence of eschar and serological tests. Prompt diagnosis and management can prevent morbidity and mortality, as it has a rapid response to doxycycline. However, due to underdiagnosis, it has often been called as the 'forgotten killer'.

Keywords: scrub typhus, neurological manifestation, meningitis, encephalitis, meningoencephalitis

1. Introduction

Scrub typhus is also known as 'tsutsugamushi disease'. It is a zoonotic disease. This disease was first mentioned in Japanese folklore to be associated with the jungle mite or 'chigger', which was named 'dangerous bug'. Therefore, the term 'tsutsugamushi' is derived from two Japanese words, 'tsutsuga' which means something small and dangerous, and 'mushi' which means creature.

'Typhus' has been derived from the Greek word 'typos' which means 'fever with stupor'. The name itself reveals a clinical aspect of the disease [1].

2. Scrub typhus

2.1. Epidemiology

Although scrub typhus was known in China in the third century A.D., it was first described by Hakuju Hashimoto in 1810 in people living in the banks of the Shinano river and later in 1879 by Baclz and Kawakami as Japanese 'flood fever'. It is widespread in the so-called 'tsutsugamushi triangle' which extends from Pakistan, India, Nepal in the West, to South Eastern Siberia, Japan, China and Korea in the North, to Indonesia, the Philippines, Northern Australia and the Pacific islands in the South. Taiwan is the centre of the tsutsugamushi triangle, and Korea has the highest reported incidence in the world [2]. About one million new cases are identified annually.

In India, the disease had occurred among troops during World War II in the state of Assam and West Bengal. Although the disease is endemic in India, epidemics have also been reported.

Epidemiological reports confirm strong existence of scrub in hilly/rain prone areas. Outbreaks reveal an autumn-winter type and a summer type of pattern. In comparison with the summer type, the autumn-winter type is less severe.

Increasing prevalence of scrub typhus reported from some Asian countries may be related to urbanization of rural areas.

2.2. Pathophysiology

Scrub typhus is caused by an obligate intracellular gram-negative bacterium called *Orientia tsutsugamushi*. Ogata in 1931 isolated the organism and named it *Rickettsia* tsutsugamushi. Now it has been renamed as *O. tsutsugamushi*. The organism lacks a cell wall. There are six important serotypes of *O. tsutsugamushi*—Gilliam, Karp, Kato, Shimokoshi, Kawasaki and Kuroki. A new strain has been isolated from a case of scrub typhus in Australia which was quite different from the classic strains and has been named as Litchfield.

The mite has four stages: egg, larva, nymph and adult. The larval forms (chiggers) transmit the disease to humans and other vertebrates. The larvae feed on rodents particularly wild rats of subgenus Rattus, The infection in humans is acquired during outdoor recreational and agricultural activities, by the bite of the larval stage of mites. The areas are usually secondary scrub growth which grows after clearance of primary forest hence the term scrub typhus. Humans are therefore accidental hosts for the pathogen. Vertical transovarial transmission occurs in mites. One case of transplacental spread has been reported in a pregnant woman, who delivered a preterm baby with scrub typhus IgM positivity.

Following the bite, the pathogen multiplies at the site of inoculation and produces both systemic and local manifestation. Infection spreads through both haematogenous and lymphatic routes. The severity of the illness depends on both host-related and pathogen-related factors. Pathogen-related factors may be related to the different strains of *O. tsutsugamushi*. Host-related factors as seen in humans with G6PD deficiency who has a worse prognosis also play a role. Target cells for multiplication are the endothelial cells of the various systems. The immune response induced by the pathogen is a combination of humoral and cell-mediated immunity. There occurs a rise of cytokines during an acute infection. There also occurs a rise in macrophage colony stimulating factor, interferon gamma and granulocyte colony stimulating factor. Therefore, the macrophage and T-lymphocyte response may be the main factor in immunity against the infection. However, the parasite has also evolved to evade the immune response of the host. The pathogen can down-regulate the expression of glycoprotein 96, in infected macrophages and endothelial

http://dx.doi.org/10.5772/intechopen.68369

cells and thereby neutralize host immune response. This molecule plays a central role antigen presentation and antibody production [3].

Central nervous system involvement occurs in scrub typhus. It is speculated that since the pathogen is an obligatory intracellular organism, it enters the cerebrospinal fluid in a monocyte or grow through the endothelium, enter via the luminal cell membrane and release into the perivascular space [4]. The pathogen also invades and multiplies in the vascular endothelium and cause wide spread vasculitis. Autopsy specimens have shown central nervous system pathology in scrub typhus cases in the form of diffuse or focal mononuclear cell infiltration of the leptomeninges, presence of typhus nodules (clusters of microglial cells) and haemorrhages of the brain substance [4].

2.3. Clinical features

The incubation period of *O. tsutsugamushi* in humans is around 10–12 days (can vary between 6 and 21 days). The clinical manifestations vary from a mild febrile illness to a severe potentially disease. The systemic features of the infection include fever, gastrointestinal disturbance, malaise, cough, myalgia and headache. A maculopapular rash starting from the trunk and spreading to the limbs is seen towards the end of the first week of the fever. Diffuse lymphadenopathy is commonly observed.

A necrotic 'eschar' at the bite site is almost diagnostic of scrub typhus (**Figure 1**).

The eschar resembles skin burn of cigarette butt. Eschar is found in 7–80% patients of scrub typhus [3]. In the authors study, eschar was detected in 28.81% of the patients of scrub typhus and 30.77% patients of meningoencephalitis due to scrub typhus [6]. The wide range of detection may be due to the difficulty in detecting eschars in dark-skinned individuals, difference in the eschar inducing capacity of the different strains of *O. tsutsugamushi*. The groin, axilla, waist and other exposed parts of the body are common sites of eschar detection. In the authors

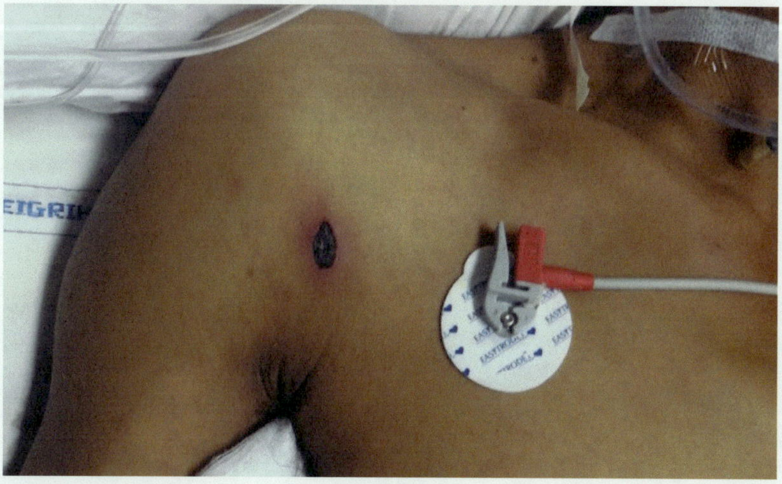

Figure 1. Eschar at bite site.

study, eschar was mostly found in the inguinal region. Different pattern of eschar distribution found in males and females due to the differences in skin folds, clothing and pressure points created by garments. The eschar not only has immense diagnostic relevance but is also important prognostically. Absence of an eschar is a risk factor for mortality [2].

Neurological involvement is often a prominent clinical manifestation of scrub typhus. However, they are still an unclear entity. Meningitis or meningoencephalitis can occur in upto one-fifth of affected patients. In the authors study, meningoencephalitis was found in 13.2% of scrub typhus patients [6]. The various neurological manifestations of scrub typhus [5] are as given in (**Table 1**).

Meningitis has features of headache, vomiting, fever, neck stiffness, along with cerebrospinal fluid (CSF) pleocytosis. Altered sensorium and fever with CSF pleocytosis are features of encephalitis. Altered sensorium with fever but normal CSF is found in encephalopathy.

Neurological manifestations in scrub typhus does not occur in isolation but are accompanied by systemic features like jaundice, breathlessness, cough, renal impairment and in some cases, with multi-organ dysfunction. In the authors study [6] neurological manifestations were associated with lymphadenopathy (46.15%), jaundice (53.85%), pulmonary oedema (23.08%), oliguria (15.38%), hepatomegaly (38.46%) and splenomegaly (7.69%). Multi-organ dysfunction was found in 15.38% patients of scrub typhus with neurological manifestation.

The most common symptom of scrub typhus is fever. The fever is usually mild and accompanied by myalgia. In the authors study the mean duration of fever was 5.61 days, prior to meningoencephalitis presentation.

Headache is a common symptom in scrub typhus (46–77%). A severe holocranial headache almost invariably occurs and thereby helps in identifying suspected cases. Headache occurs

Direct involvement
1. Meningitis
2. Meningoencephalitis
3. Encephalitis
4. Encephalopathy
5. Seizure
6. Stroke
Immune mediated
1. Optic neuritis
2. Myelitis
3. Acute-disseminated encephalomyelitis
4. Neuropathy

Table 1. Neurological involvement in scrub typhus.

http://dx.doi.org/10.5772/intechopen.68369

not only in patients of meningitis or meningoencephalitis but in other scrub typhus patients also. However, in those cases, the headache is less severe.

In scrub typhus meningitis, the severe headache is associated with neck stiffness and fever. Other signs of meningeal irritation like Kernig's sign may also be present. These meningeal signs are detected in upto 45% patients. In the author's study, meningeal signs were present in 76.92% patients [6].

Altered sensorium is present in scrub typhus patient with encephalitis and meningoencephalitis. In the author's study, altered sensorium was found in all patients; however, other studies have reported a lower incidence.

Seizure occurs in scrub typhus with neurological involvement in 22–50% cases, though uncommon myoclonic seizure was found in one patient in the author's series.

Cranial nerve deficits are seen in 25% patients. Most commonly sixth nerve involvement is seen, which maybe unilateral or bilateral. Facial palsy may occur in isolation or in association with Guillain Barre syndrome [2]. Cochlear nerve involvement occurs in about 19% patients and cause sensorineural hearing loss, otalgia and tinnitus. This may be due to direct invasion by the pathogen or due to a secondary immune-mediated effect.

Other uncommon neurological manifestations of scrub typhus mentioned are infarction, cerebellitis, haemorrhages, subdural hematoma and Guillain Barre syndrome [2].

2.4. Diagnosis of scrub typhus

This is aided by serological tests in appropriate clinical setting.

Microimmunofluorescence is considered the test of choice. However, lack of fluorescent microscopes makes it difficult for most hospitals.

Latex agglutination, indirect haemagglutination, immunoperoxidase assay, ELISA and polymerase chain reaction (PCR) are also available. The nested PCR is more sensitive than the serological tests.

PCR can be used to detect rickettsial DNA in both blood and eschar samples. The PCR is targeted at the gene encoding the major 56-kDa antigen and/or 47-kDa surface antigen gene. The results are best within first week for blood samples.

ELISA (IgG and IgM) technique, particularly immunoglobulin M (IgM), capture assays are probably the most sensitive test available for rickettsial diagnosis. In cases of infection with *O. tsutsugamushi*, a significant IgM antibody titre is observed at the end of the first week, whereas IgG antibodies appear at the end of the second week.

Weil Felix test: the sharing of the antigen between rickettsia and proteus is the basis of this heterophile antibody test. Though this test lacks high sensitivity and specificity, it is inexpensive. The test should be carried out after 5–7 days of onset of fever.

However, due to the antigenic diversity of the pathogen, a battery of tests may be required for the diagnosis [1].

CSF analysis in scrub typhus meningoencephalitis reveals mild-to-moderate elevation in protein, low-to-normal glucose and mild degree of lymphocytic pleocytosis. By using nested PCR, the genotypes invading the central nervous system (CNS) may be identified. By this, it was suggested that the Karp and Boryong genotypes possibly invade the CNS more than other types [4]. In the author's study, tuberculous meningitis remained the close differential diagnosis of scrub typhus meningitis due to similar CSF findings [6]. However, CSF adenosine deaminase (ADA) may be helpful, as it is elevated >10 in tuberculous meningitis, unlike scrub typhus meningitis.

Neurological involvement in scrub typhus is usually associated with a normal MRI and non-specific EEG slowing. Often MRI of brain in scrub typhus may reveal features of ischemic changes due to vasculitis or parainfectious demyelination [5].

2.5. Treatment

Doxycycline is the drug of choice. It is bacteriostatic to *O. tsutsugamushi* but does not cross the blood brain barrier beyond 15–30% [2]. Therefore, in some instances, neurological deterioration can continue despite doxycycline therapy. This may be due to resistance, immune-mediated injury, or due to drug interactions with oral antacids. Doxycycline is given in the dose of 200 mg/day, in two divided doses, for individuals above 45 kgs body weight, for a duration of 7 days. In children, doxycycline is given in the dose of 4.5 mg/kg body weight in two divided doses. Doxycycline is contraindicated in pregnant women. In complicated cases, intravenous is given followed by oral doxycycline to complete 7–15 days of therapy.

Azithromycin is another drug which can be used in a dose of 500 mg daily for 5 days and 10 mg/kg body weight in children for 5 days. It can also be given intravenously in complicated cases. Azithromycin is the drug of choice in pregnant women with scrub typhus. It is also preferred in patients of scrub typhus with renal failure, where doxycycline is not given.

In complicated cases, Chloramphenicol can also be used. It is administered intravenously at a dose of 50–100 mg/kg/day, 6 hourly doses, followed by oral therapy to complete 7–15 days of therapy.

Doxycycline and/or chloramphenicol resistant strains have been detected in South-East Asia. These strains are sensitive to Azithromycin.

Patients with meningoencephalitis due to scrub typhus can be additionally administered with dexamethasone, or mannitol, if they have altered sensorium or cranial nerve deficits.

Recovery is usually brisk with appropriate therapy.

Pre-antibiotic era mortality was more than 60%; however, recent data show a mortality of approximately 30% [2]. In the author's study [6], the mortality was 15.38%. Mortality is usually associated with multi-organ dysfunction syndrome.

3. Conclusion

Neurological complication is not uncommon in scrub typhus. They present with acute febrile illness with altered sensorium and meningeal signs. The presence of 'eschar' helps in early diagnosis, but they are often absent. Prompt CSF analysis is required on clinical suspicion of neurological features in scrub typhus patients. Timely initiation of therapy results in recovery and less complications.

Author details

Masaraf Hussain

Address all correspondence to: masarafhussain@yahoo.co.in

Department of Neurology, North Eastern Indira Gandhi Regional Institute of Health and Medical Sciences, Shillong, India

References

[1] Mahajan SK. Scrub typhus. JAPI. Nov 2005;Vol. **53**:954-957

[2] Vishwanath S, Muthu V, Iqbal N, Bhavith R. Scrub typhus meningitis in South India-A retrospective study. PLOS ONE. /www.plosone.org June 2013/Volume 8/Issue 6/e66595

[3] Rajapakse S, Rodrigo C, Fernando D. Asian Pacific Journal of Tropical Medicine. April 2012;Vol. 5(Issue 4):253-57

[4] Pai H, Sohn S, Scong Y. Central nervous system involvement in patients with scrub typhus. Clinical Infectious Diseases. 1997;**24**:436-440

[5] Jamil MD, Hussain M, Lyngdoh M, Sharma S, Barman B. Scrub typhus meningoencephalitis, a diagnostic challenge for clinicians: A hospital based study from North East India. Journal of Neuroscience in Rural Practice. 2015;Vol. **6**(Issue 4):488-493. DOI: 10.4103/0976-3147.169769

[6] Misra UK, Kalita J, Mani VE. Neurological manifestations of scrub typhus. Journal of Neurology, Neurosurgery, and Psychiatry. 2015;**86**:761-766